A MOMENT GONE

S. Westwood

S. Westwood

Published by
Chipmunkapublishing
PO Box 6872
Brentwood
Essex CM13 1ZT
United Kingdom

http://www.chipmunkapublishing.com

Front cover art by Ashley Westwood, photography Juliet Morris

Chipmunkapublishing gratefully acknowledge the support of Arts Council England.

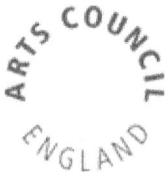

A Moment Gone

For Lydia Angel, much loved and never forgotten x

S. Westwood

A Moment Gone

Introduction

Writing is cathartic, whether it be autobiographical or not. My first novel 'Suicide Junkie' aired all my dirty laundry to the public gaze and deciding to write it was not an easy decision. I guess the main reason I wrote it was to get it out of me, to get all those awful things that happened out of my mind so that I could put them away. I can now put all that behind me in a book on my shelf. I had always written and always wanted to have a book published so it fulfilled a dream, but after it was published I realised it was much more important than I had given it credit for. It had turned fifteen years of suffering into something positive and, most importantly, helped others. I have become a spokesperson for raising awareness of BDD - body Dysmorphic disorder, the mental illness I suffered with since I was fifteen and, although very much better, I still suffer to this day. I have had my story in magazines and have appeared on TV talking about my experience with the disorder and hopefully making it more well known. Hopefully helping people.

So what is BDD? Basically it is perceived ugliness. But more than a normal appearance concern it takes over every aspect of your life. It is obsessing over a small or nonexistent flaw in your appearance to such a degree that it disables you in many ways and causes deep depression. I had it to such an extent that I attempted suicide many times. BDD was not my only reason for suicide, it is seldom just one thing that leads you down that path, but BDD is very difficult to live with. The worst thing about it for me was that I didn't know the problem was mental. I knew that I obsessed over my looks too much but I felt so hideously ugly that I could not help but obsess. I would spend hours in front of the mirror putting on make up and picking at my skin. I would go from room to room checking my appearance in every reflective surface, walking around with a mirror held in front of my face hoping that in a different light I might look acceptable. If only I had seen someone on TV talking about these symptoms I might have realised that I had it too, that my skin wasn't red and flawed, that it was all in my mind.

So that is my mission. To at least get through to one person that is in that dark place that I was. I think I have achieved that. Since having my book published in December 06 I have spent my time promoting it, taking part in training days to educate Gps, teachers, people in the mental health world about suicide, self harm and BDD. Public speaking at these events and on TV and radio. Doing something worthwhile.

During a talk about recovery I said that I was 70% better and that the other 30% I had just learnt to live with. I still have bad days but I cope with them better than I used to. A lot of my strength comes from Ashley, my wife of three years. Without her I don't know how those percentages might change. I also made the decision to not work a nine to five job anymore. That was a step into the dark but I have done work in the past year that is so much more rewarding. I could not bear all those hours alone with my thoughts, thinking of suicide instead of looking for a missing t shirt. My job

A Moment Gone

seemed so futile. Recovery doesn't mean that you have gone back to doing what you were doing before. I don't ever want to go back to that sort of work because it made me so ill. Yet I am at a stage in recovery that means I can do other things that only a few years ago would have been impossible. How could I go on TV when I found it impossible to even leave the house? Well, medication is helping me a lot, but I am helping me a lot as well.

Wanting to get better is not as natural as it seems. I wanted so badly to not have BDD. But my depression I still cling to like a security blanket. I understand myself as a depressed male. All my artistic flare comes out when I am low. As some shiny happy person I would be lost. But I guess I'll never be one of those- I will always have attempted suicide, I will always know what that feels like. Now I have a wife and a son I have to give in to the fact that suicide is not an option anymore, and that is hard. Where can I turn to when I get those feelings back? And those self harming and self neglectful feelings are still there, they are merely repressed and I am almost certain that if I was on my own I would be a wreck. I need to have people relying on me because I can't rely on myself. But I more than anyone know how life can change. You do not know what life holds so better hold it close.

So, that is who I am, that is where I am, a recovering plane crash that frets at the future and clings to the present as it is as far as I can see. I used to cling to the past, but now I use it. I would not be me without those past events, I often think how much better it would have been if I had always been with Ashley, but perhaps that wouldn't have worked. If I had met her before I had begun recovery I may well have pushed her away. If I hadn't had some bad relationships I would not have learnt how to have a good one. We are who we are from the things we have done and the things we have thought. There is no point wishing the past away. Our souls are grown, they are not given to us whole. Mine has been shaped by events and the feelings that came from it. And the only way I could voice that transition was to write.

So what is this book? This book is part of my past that I wish to accept in my future. It is not always as negative as I was back then. Each story reflects a frame of mind that saw how much better things could be yet struggled to find them. I wrote stories to explain, however cryptically, my own thoughts. I wrote fables, perhaps sometimes even children's stories with moral meanings geared to help the reader to learn the lessons I have had to learn. Perhaps one of my stories will hit a chord and make sense of something. I have had to make sense of a lot. Some of these stories are just that, they are stories, ideas I have had and wanted to put down, writing because I love the medium and I have to do it. Writing when doing anything else seemed pointless. I even entered one of my stories in to a local short story competition. 'Your time will come' had already been written but as it was fairly positive I sent it in. I won first prize and for a while I felt pretty good about my writing. It was not long after that little ego boost that I decided to take my writing seriously. Sometimes I think I can write, other times I feel I am wasting my time. That is just my negativity. No art is a waste of time. Even the

A Moment Gone

stories that are simple tales reflect where my mind was. A hopeless romantic, a gothic depressive with a love for words. And these are my words. Written in various stages of distress. Some were written on computer, some were scribbled on a page, some passages were even written at work on yellow post it notes. I hope they are of interest, I hope they help, inspire or merely pass some time. These are my words.

S.Westwood.

S. Westwood

A Moment Gone

The Walk

He walks along the road he has always walked- the road which will lead him home. But he is in no rush to reach his destination, for this walk is important. The things in his mind must work themselves through before he reaches his door. But there are so many things; so much has been said. His mind struggles to keep it all together.

His legs move without his brain having to signal to them. His brain has better things to do. His mind is a thought, and there is room for nothing else. The road goes on travelling under his feet. Cars travel past and pay him no mind. It is only inside him that the insanity shows like a firework display of emotion.

Rain comes, darkness of clouds that should dull the mind. But the gentle drops of water falling upon his head make no impact. He does not even notice, and his legs keep up that same steady pace.

The rain does not like to be ignored, and so it comes down faster, heavier, wetter. His hair falls, soaked down over his eyes. His clothes cling, cold to his body. Yet he walks, his mind thinks, and nothing outside of his frame means anything to him.

Let his house move away from him. As he walks, let his home move also. Let the road grow and have no end. Let the rain come and the wind blow. There will never be time for his thoughts to settle, so let him just keep on walking. He is always walking.

A Spell Of Love

In her room the light of the last candle dims into darkness, and then her eyes adjust to see once more. She sits on her bed, back on the pillow and legs stretched out in front of her. She has been that way for hours, staring forwards, looking at the door. She has been that way ever since he left. She had no idea she would feel so empty without him filling the room. She had no idea that she would have to live through this moment. This time was never supposed to come.

He had gone through that door; he had let it fall half closed, and there it stayed. Somewhere far distant from those four walls, he went on with his life while hers was as still as death. If only he had blessed her with that release. He had surely taken away her life, yet somehow her heart continued to beat, and her lungs went on breathing. Such pain should have killed her, yet there she was, and there she would stay.

Let the weight fall from her bones. Let her stomach starve and shrivel into nothing. Let her mouth dry up and set still. Let her bones sit and look at that door; let her corpse wait for his return. For it would take that long, and she knew it. He was not coming back to her.

How many had he touched in this way? That phantom, drifting into existence's from out of the cold night. Coming into the warmth of a home and into the warmth of the bed. The touch of yielding female flesh under the grip of his huge hands and agile serpent fingers.

"Can I fetch you something my sweet?

A Moment Gone

Before I come to you."

His words were still within that room, playing amidst the dust in the air. And the remembered visions of him were dancing with the shadows. Such a beauty he was, like no man should be, for such beauty is dangerous in the hands of a male. It was a female's beauty, a pure exquisiteness, as perfect as a sculpture and just as pale. Yet he was handsome not pretty. A man chiseled from fine white marble and then lovingly smoothed. A man who had borrowed his lips from the cherubs and his eyes from the blue waters of the sea. Dark eyebrows and hair that moved gently in the breeze as he stepped up to the door.

He knocked, and he waited. His face fell into peace, his eyelids resting before they opened. And she had gone to him, to meet her stranger at the door.

"I am sorry to disturb you, but my car seems to have given up the ghost, and I can't find a phone box around. Could I possibly…"

She had invited him in, for she knew who he was; he with those eyes that looked right into her body and soul. He with the sweet voice of a thousand whispers becoming a whole. He who's body moved beneath that jacket, promising a handsome nakedness.

She had been waiting for him, and she had brought him into her house.

Such an effect he had on her, the strength of it took her by surprise. The sum of his parts added up to twice what they would in any other man. But this was the man she had dreamt of for so many years. This was her creation manifest from all those vivid, lucid dreams. Dreams full of sweetness and light. Dreams of him coming to her, and coming with her in sex that filled a hunger no food ever could; a thirst no water could reach; and an ache that only his touch could soothe.

This was how it was supposed to be, yet it had felt so strange. How could she love him so without the slightest knowledge of his life? Why was she so willing to give him everything that was her and ask for as little in return as a single kiss? It was such strange magic that it scared her.

She had been excited as a child when she heard the knock at the door, quickly applying more lipstick before going to him. A brief look at herself in the mirror, a smile on her face; she could not believe she was so lucky to have this chance.

She opened the door and swooned at the sight of him. Even her imagination had not been able to piece together something as wonderful as he. She had no idea of the feelings the mere sight of him would invoke.

Years ago, as a child, she had dreamt of a man with such beauty and with such words:

"I do not wish to step out of line, but you really are amazingly beautiful."

She had smiled at his flattery, and smiled to herself. He had no idea; he probably never did; yet this was his life, and this was his purpose. She had done nothing wrong, merely calling upon he that was, surely, always meant for her anyway. Yet there was a price to pay, there always is. For every happiness, nature must even it with pain. For every corruption of nature, there must then be balance, and pain will soon tip the scales.

A Moment Gone

One stolen night she had. One night which lasted for the shortest forever. Arms around her, lips on hers, flesh within flesh. Kisses and caresses sending sensations to every part of her long deserted body.

But it was over now. He left at dawn. He left as surely as the night leaves to let in the day. But he was not coming back.

She should have known it really. She should have known that it would only last for one glorious night. But she had taken that risk. She had read from that book and she had mixed her herbs. She had called on him to come to her. The magic was so basic and so slight. And the spell had worked, but the magic had died. Soon it would be her turn.

S. Westwood

You're so beautiful. Those eyes that shine right
into me and see who I am.
No lies.
A precious face, to me, worth a thousand trees, a
million tropical sunsets.
A soul more beautiful than nature bestows its
beauty on the birds and the animals.
I am lost. There is no way back.
Nothing else is beautiful anymore.

A Moment Gone

A Girl With A Blade Of Grass

If she stared at it any longer her eyes would phase and turn green, lost in its colour. She did not care what she might look like to other people, sitting there with a single blade of grass held up between two fingers, the breeze gently rocking it South. She did not care that she had looked at it for such a long time that her eyes had blurred. Just let it speak to her again, as it had done a moment ago. Let it speak and prove that she was not completely crazy.

She shook it, and she stared at it a little angrily.

"Come on," she spoke, as if calling a cat in for the night, "come on, speak..." She was losing her patience.

The blade of grass fell down over her finger, no longer strong enough to hold itself upright through all this interrogation. Stupid thing, playing with her like that. She had not asked it to speak in the first place.

Earlier that day her mother had scolded her for the fifth time that week, each time for simple childish naughtiness. Since when had it been a crime to be a child anyway? A mother should know that she is not going to give birth to an adult. Well, the fifth time was one too many, and Mary had run away.

There were a lot of places to run to where she lived, but none seemed so attractive as the meadow behind her house. At the end of her garden a fence kept the real nature out as it turned into a hill of grass, daises and buttercups. Such freedom it offered, and that is where she had run to, running over the brow of the hill to become hidden on the other side. She doubted that her mother would find her there, despite how obvious the hiding place was; it was just too easy.

Her mother was cruel to her, so Mary wanted to punish her with worry. She had been in her garden for mere minutes before the thought struck her to leave. She would run away, and then they would be sorry for all the things they said. She would run away and let nature take care of her.

As soon as she had got there, she fell down into the soft arms of the grass and broke into giggles as the ends of it tickled her skin. The bright sun soaked into her face and reflected upon the white of her lace-frilled dress. And the harsh words of her mother were lost in the gentle caress of a thousand grass blades. And then there was that one- that special one.

As she lay with her head on its side, she stared at a single blade of grass, smiling at its perfection. It glowed with its colour, proud to be so green and natural, standing erect and pointing to the sky that gave it light. It stood there and faced her; it stood there and spoke:

"Don't worry Mary, your mother loves you really."

Her smile dropped with shock. She was paralysed with doubt. And if you have never heard grass speak before, then you will understand how surprising this was. Its voice was so sweet that she was not even able to feel afraid.

"You are loved Mary."

She sat up now, with eyes still firmly fixed to

A Moment Gone

the blade of grass, from which she was sure the voice had come. Nothing. It did not move, nor did it speak any words to comfort her shock. It was just there; it was just grass.

For a time she sat there waiting, half expecting it to speak again, to move and to come alive, but it did none of those things. It was grass and it stood as grass always stands, one of so many that make up the green of the hill. It was nothing but a fragment of the meadow's mosaic. Yet it had spoken had it not?

She bent down, holding it between her fingers, and plucked it from the ground. There was a little noise as it snapped free, and then another misplaced sound that resembled a faint, pitiful scream.

Mary sat and listened, but heard no more. That was it- and no amount of coaxing would make it speak again. It lay in the palm of her hand now, as lifeless as it ought to be, and when the breeze came strong enough to take it from her, that was it, it was lost, it was gone.

Your mother loves you really....

Yes, she thought, I suppose she does. She was just being a mother, just as she was being a daughter, and that was how it was meant to be. Her mother loved her, and Mary loved her too.

And so she left the beautiful meadow, she left the hill, she left the grass to be the grass, and she went back home to be a child.

S. Westwood

A moment, gone
A hope, lost
A chance, mistaken.
A reason?
For what?
Everything I ever wanted.

A Moment Gone

Curfew

In this day and age, life is more certain, that is to say, death is less ambiguous. There is an order to things, a time scale to everything. There are no old people draining the government of money. There are no homes keeping the elderly alive, waiting for when they will die. There are no bus passes or coach trips to Eastbourne. But how do we feel about all this, really?

People cope in different ways, but no one is free of it. The president, the MPs and the doctors employed to implant the chips in the first place- no one is spared the fate of dying on their fortieth birthday. The electronic chip, placed in the brain at the moment of birth, timed and primed with poison, let into the blood stream at exactly forty years of life. It sends some people mad, but it gives some people clarity.

I remember a story about a family who knew one of the doctors. They paid him a fortune to put his job on the line, and to risk imprisonment, so that he would implant the chip in their new-born son without arming it. At forty years old that child should have died; he didn't, but his fate was still certain. He became insane with paranoia, waiting for the government to find him, and he hung himself within a few months of that birthday.

Suicide is high. Many see no point in living at all when death is so certain- but has death not always been certain? Putting a time on us has some strange effects in the physique. Many kill themselves at thirty-nine, just to prove that they can still control their own fate. Some live the life of a libertine, trying to get in as much fun as possible and often die young through all their excesses. Others struggle with achievement, hoping to at least leave some mark on the world to prove that they were once here.

Has this improved things? Is it right that we are born into a death sentence? Is it right to have a law enforced that sends so many people insane with fear, cutting into their own skulls, trying to remove the chip, fighting to survive as all animals do?

I myself am happy to know how long I have. I am pleased that I do not have to save money for a day when I will be too frail to work, and to ill too spend it. I am glad that I am surrounded in beauty and do not have to look upon the ravages of time in the wrinkled faces of the old. I would hate to think that, one-day, I will lose my ability to function and that others would have to care for me.

This was, really, the only answer to solving the over population problems on a planet, straining under our weight. At least we all have enough food to eat and water to drink. At least we can walk and breathe clean air.

I am twenty-nine; I have eleven years left. The government is currently in talks about dropping the age of life to thirty. But I am safe; I have eleven years before my chip expires, and I will live to see my son reach fifteen.

A Moment Gone

Worlds Join

The town was in darkness, but here there were orbs of light in which people sat and talked beneath the warm red glow of outside heaters. Each table had its own light, its own heat, its own little populated world.

Four souls sat there on wooden stalls, arms rested on the wooden table, hands hovering close to their glasses of wheat scented beer or sweet flavoured spirits. Four people engulfed in the gentle glow of light, secluded from all others by the veil of night time black and by the fact that all others were strangers and all others had their own worlds to be part of. This was theirs. Their eyes were only interested in the faces of those so close to them, their ears only hearing the words each other was speaking. Their world.

She had been there, at that table, for the last half an hour, feeling that lovely warmth given out by the burning gas in that beacon like heater. She was there amongst the others, listening to their conversations and listening to their laughter.

People always laughed in these places. She could hear that sound all around her coming from those other tables, those other worlds. And if you try hard you can adjust your ears to hear their distant words as well. You could pin point a voice, home in on it, and hear what it says. That is what she had done a little earlier, and that was why she had decided to join these people.

She already knew the names of those that sat around her: Simon, Paul, Darren and Anthony. She knew because she listened, and she knew them because she actually heard what they said with their mouths, and looked into their eyes to hear what they did not say. She knew what they wanted, and she knew which of them needed it more.

Moments before she had been at a different table, a world just to the left of this one. She had been there, listening to the people in the very same way as she was doing now. She had heard Lucy's words and she had heard her thoughts. She had understood more than any of those loving friends that surrounded her. Or was it that her friends knew it too, but knew they could do nothing to help? Well she could…

It was time for action. With one energetic leap she jumped onto the table. All those young men sitting around her were startled.

Paul put his hand to his heart.

"Bloody cat nearly gave me a heart attack. Get rid of it Simon, flea ridden thing."

"Awww, leave it alone," Simon said and stroked her soft ginger fur. She purred and rubbed her head up against the palm of his hand. "It's lovely."

Simon was the one, and she had known that from the first moment she heard his voice. Now it was time for stage two. She walked daintily to the edge of the table and sat there looking ahead into the darkness. Simon's attention never left her, and he was observing her behavior with much curiosity.

Then he followed the cat's gaze, looking past the darkness and over to the table that was on their left. That was what the cat appeared to be staring at. He looked on, searched, adjusted his

A Moment Gone

blurry vision and saw, under the light, a face he thought that he recognised.

At that very moment the cat pushed forwards, landed safely on the ground, and then walked slowly over to the other table. Simon still watched in growing fascination and by that time had put a name to the face...It was Lucy.

The cat leapt up onto the other table and Lucy proceeded to stroke her just like Simon had done. Lucy...a girl Simon had once known, a girl he thought was lost forever.

It took a few moments before anxiety gave way to what he felt he had to do. He got up and moved towards her, seeing her clearer and remembering all the more. He was uneasy at first, yet determined all the same, moving away from his own small world to go and join in hers.

"Lucy?"

She looked at him, kind blue eyes sparkled and a huge smile filled her petite face.

"Simon!" Her voice was thankfully full of happy surprise.

The cat continued to rub its head on Lucy's hand despite the fact that she had stopped stroking it and was looking only at Simon. But the cat knew what was happening. The cat knew that something had begun. And, because it was the only noise it was able to make, it let out a soft meow.

Lucy looked back down at the pretty ginger cat and stroked it again with a smile that never wanted to leave.

"It's a lovely cat isn't it?" Simon said.

"Yes she's beautiful." Lucy answered. And then she addressed the cat: "What's your name then?" And she began to try uncovering the name tag that hung from its collar, hiding under thick ginger fur.

"What is it?" Simon asked as Lucy held the little gold tag in her fingers.

"Her name's Cupid." She said.

A Moment Gone

Her Release

They say she was beautiful and had a heart of gold, but I knew it wasn't true. If her heart were stone then she would not have bled so bad. She was beautiful though, once. I saw dreams in her eyes, but they say she kept her thoughts in a book by her bed. Such lies they told. And whenever did a corpse smell of strawberries? But that is what I remember, the open coffin in that room, scented like sweet fruit.

I can close my eyes and be there, seeing her lying peacefully, a doll with eyelids that close when you put it down. But then I open my eyes again, and I remember how I saw her that night, covered in blood, the heart that once beat so close to mine now no longer beating at all.

And they said that Lucy killed herself, but I knew she would never leave me. But then, why was she there, crushed by the ground that caught her fall? Something about it made no sense, but I could make sense of something. She was gone, wherever that was. She was not here anymore.

And so I will follow her, because she never could escape me. When she slept I was in her dreams, and I was in her bed. When she cried the tears were bitter sweet and tasted like love. Her whole body tasted like that.

I would not be able to live without holding that body again. I would not be able to live with the memory of it in my mind, and all those accusing words and trials.

Lucy, your father is coming to find you...be good to daddy.

S. Westwood

The Hesitant Frog

The frog sat at the water's edge and stared at its own reflection in the ripples. The pond was dirty and full of plant life that took up so much of the space. And even though it was hot outside the water was not so very tempting. How would he see to swim in such a murky place? How could he avoid getting himself caught in those clouds of thick algae? The only thing the water served at that moment was a perfect mirror in which he could see himself.

A fine frog he was. Not so long ago he was nothing but a black, legless creature, just a head with a tail. Now look at him- he had come so far. He was a light shade of green with unique black markings over his smooth body. His legs were fully-grown and tucked to his side, ready to propel him with an energetic jump. But he sat still. He was a frog, whether he was swimming, or whether he sat; it was what he was.

Somewhere near the middle of the pond a few bubbles made way for the head of a fellow frog just breaking the surface as he came up for air. His large eyes caught sight of the frog sitting on the bank, and he spoke.

"What are you doing sitting there?"

The young frog was startled to have been addressed, yet he answered straight away.

"Just sitting, and thinking."

"Well why aren't you coming into the pond?"

"Well," the young frog said while he thought, "I know this bank- I crawled up here as soon as my legs had grown and I've got used to the feel of dry

A Moment Gone

dirt between my toes. I have no idea what is in that water."

"But it's a frog's instinct to be in the water, don't you feel that?" The other frog asked sounding concerned for his new friend.

"Well yes; I know that I should be in there, but what need have I to change where I am? I know this place, so why go into somewhere unknown?"

The frog in the middle of the pond looked rather puzzled, but then began to swim to the edge. The young frog watched him swim and reach him at the bank.

"It's wonderful here," the other frog said. "This is the life for a frog."

"I have been there once you know, when I was younger…I nearly got eaten."

"But you are bigger now, this is where you should be."

"Do not worry for me," the young frog smiled, "it frightens me to change. I will be fine here."

The older frog trod water for a few moments looking at the young and beautiful frog that sat on the edge. But he had spoken as many words as he could find, and if he could not convince him, then he had tried his best. In time, he decided to leave. The air was good for a moment, but he had no intention of making it a habit.

The young frog watched as his new friend disappeared under the water, and he sat as he had before, staring at the ripples, only slightly phased by the conversation and by the fact that he was alone once again.

Secretly, he wished that he could be in the

water.   Secretly, it was only his fear that kept him on the surface.   And sitting there, on his own, his body began to dry and harden.   His body took in the sun, and his body broke.   Sitting there, alone, he died.

A Moment Gone

Another Suicide

Your funeral
The last chance to see all your friends,
Friends you did not even know you had.
But you do not see
And you never have
And this last good-bye
You cannot give.

But those you leave behind feel sorry.
Those you follow all regret.

If only you had given more time,
Or if only you had been given more time
From them,
Maybe things could have changed.

But your mind always incarcerated your happiness
in a cage that it could never escape from,
And the people around you hurt you with their
smiles.

You thought that no one cared,
Perhaps they didn't,
But how will you ever know…now?

S. Westwood

The Old Oval Mirror

Mona awoke as the alarm clock rang painfully in her ears. With an outstretched arm she found the off button and the noise ceased. As always it was a rude awakening one hour before she had to be at work. She squashed her face into the pillow wanting just a few minutes more comfort before she had to confront the bathroom. But she knew that the time was stolen, she knew that if she was not careful she would fall back to sleep and then she would have to call in sick. Better to not go in to work at all than to be late and if she did not get her usual hour of preparation time she could not function.

She sat up and swung her bare legs over the side of the bed catching her reflection in the tall mirror on the wardrobe door. What a state she thought. Her shoulder length brown hair was matted at the back and she looked old and tired. She stood as she stared at herself, her red satin night dress falling back down over her knees. Her brown eyes seemed almost black and lacked life; dark circles underneath made it look like she had not slept in days. Old at thirty-five.

She dragged herself into the bathroom and lifted the night-dress over her head, throwing it down on the floor. God! Why did she insist on having mirrors in the house? She had caught sight of her reflection again, an unwanted image of her naked body, its curves in all the wrong places, shadows proving that she had too much flesh, or too much fat. She averted her gaze and faced the shower. She still had time to make herself look

A Moment Gone

something close to human.

Mona took a shower and then went back to the bedroom to fix her wet hair. She had a routine and she always stuck to it. Drying and combing her hair and then applying a layer of make up to hide her face. She hated what she looked like, she hated having to look at herself and sometimes she would be late for work because something had gone wrong. Perhaps she would have a blemish, perhaps the make up had not hidden everything and she would be thrown into a state of panic. It wasn't vanity, it was fear. No one ever saw Mona without her 'war paint'.

And then she had to face the public. She worked as a cashier at the local supermarket. Smiling and saying 'morning' or 'afternoon' to the shoppers that would often not give her so much as a nod. They were probably looking at her thinking bad things. Thinking that they were better than her because they were not mere shop assistants. Thinking how fat and ugly she was. She served them all with her professional courtesy, yet wishing so much that she could be one of them. They all had such good skin. They were all so much slimmer and probably had great careers. She was doomed to always be nothing.

At the end of her shift she went through the staff room to get her bag and coat from the locker. There were three of the girls in there, all six eyes staring at Mona as she went passed. She heard them snigger and then one of them spoke.

"Wish I was finishing now."

Mona did not look up feeling exposed now that eyes were on her as she unlocked the grey metal locker, pulling out her coat and sending her bag falling to the floor. She knew they were all looking at her, she knew what they must be thinking. She put her coat on and did it up before leaning down to retrieve her bag.

"You found yourself a man yet Mona?" One of the girls asked. But Mona knew that it was not so much a question as an all too familiar taunt. She did not answer but walked briskly towards the door with her head hung low, leaving them to their boastful conversations about the men in their lives and the fabulous clothes that they wore. Mona was not part of that world; no man would ever want her now; she had been single for six years.

As she left the room she literally bumped in to Brenda in the doorway.

"Sorry" Brenda said and for a moment looked as though she were waiting for Mona to speak. An uncomfortable silence was soon broken. "Are you coming out with the girls tomorrow night?"

Mona knew that the girls had arranged a night out at the pub and it seemed that all of them in turn had asked her if she was coming. Why would they not leave her alone? She had no intention of going. What use was she to a party? She would only get in the way. People would talk to her because they would feel sorry for her and she would have to try and talk with nothing whatsoever to say. And it was safer to not make plans. All too often Mona had said that she would be somewhere and her face had let her down. If she could not get the make up right she would not be able to go. People would look at her, people would stare at her terrible complexion. Safer to

A Moment Gone

stay at home with her TV screen and a face pack on, fearing a knock at the door. Fearing that they would know she was in despite the fact that she was hiding behind the sofa.

"I don't know yet," Mona answered feeling uncomfortable, and with that she lowered her head and left.

Outside was dark and cold, winter in all its gloom, the release of Christmas long forgotten. One security light lit the place where she had parked but her car was not in the spotlight. It didn't feel safe in the staff car park all alone and Mona walked briskly to the little red Micra and got in it as quickly as possible. Before long she was on the journey home.

Mona lived alone with only her cat Frizz for company. Her last boyfriend had cheated on her with her best friend and now both of them were out of her life. That was six years ago and she had still not gotten over it, she probably never would. She had not had another boyfriend or made a single friend since. A cat is more loyal. A cat 's love is unconditional. A cat is wild yet it chooses to come home, and every time that Frizz came back, Mona was honored. The cat was not waiting on the doorstep of the flat when Mona arrived.

The next day was Saturday and, after a lie in, Mona had decided to go to the antique shops in Anchor Place. She liked going there, an arcade of little antique stores crammed full with treasures from times past. It had a 1920's feel with old music playing and models garbed in sequined dresses, tiny handbags under their arms. It was one of Mona's favorite places to visit and somewhere that she could enjoy alone.

Mona left the flat at eleven and the cat never had come back home. Mona was a touch concerned but it was not completely out of character. Mona thought deeply as she went to her car, 'if I was her I wouldn't want to come home to me either.'

The antique arcade always got Mona quite excited. As she entered she was instantly taken back in time and her chest tightened in anticipation. Antique furniture filled the first of the shops, dark and light glossy wood, cabinets with carved spiral struts, writing desks with all their little drawers and secret compartments. Mona was in her element. She loved all these old and beautiful things, she had no time for modernism. If only her shop assistant wage allowed her the extravagance her taste called for. She would surround herself in all those wonderful objects and she could stay inside forever just looking at them.

There were glass cabinets all around with trinkets; ornaments and jewellery. Shops decked out as though they were rooms in some stately home, lamps in the corner with stained glass shades. So much to take in, so refreshingly different to the supermarket where she spent most of her waking hours. If only she could drown herself in nostalgia.

As she entered the last shop she caught sight of something familiar yet so different that she was caught unawares in shock. It was her reflection! She gasped and held her heart in exclamation.

There, in front of her was an old oval mirror,

A Moment Gone

its frame a dark metal carved in ornate spirals, its glass large enough to reflect Mona's entire upper body. But what she was looking at was all wrong. It was her face, her features, yet she was utterly beautiful!

She went slowly towards it, watching herself getting closer, the image in the mirror growing in detail yet the nearer she was the more lovely she looked. There were no lines from age, there was no plumpness to her body or to her cheeks, there was no blemish on her face. It looked almost as if she was in soft focus, her features making up a film star pose her hair falling in perfect highlighted ringlets. Was it her at all? What illusion was this?

"Very special mirror that." A man's voice came from behind her. She was startled by the sudden noise but did not look around. She just looked deeper into her own face, a face she had always dreamt of having and a face that was hers.

"Could do with a clean mind," the man continued, "but yours for twenty."

Mona was paralysed, almost afraid, but was she scared to be so happy? It was as if a key had been turned, a lock that was always keeping Mona from the world, but now she had escaped.

"I'll take it." She said, and finally she managed to stop looking at her own ravishing beauty and turned to see the short, suited shop keeper. "Yes, I'll take it please."

When Mona arrived home Frizz was waiting. She carried the mirror into the flat and the cat coiled around her legs purring loudly. She leant the mirror against the hallway wall and went to the kitchen to feed her.

"Now what to do Frizz?" She asked the cat as she put its bowl down in front of its expectant face. "I'll take the others down, yes that's what I'll do."

And so Mona went in to the bathroom and went straight to the mirror that hung on the far wall. She did not make eye contact with it, afraid to break the illusion that her new find had achieved, but lifted it free and turned it around leaving the room and discarding the mirror in the hall. Frizz was not eating but following her every move, getting under her feet. Mona went back to the kitchen and searched the drawer for a screwdriver. The tool belonged to her ex. She had inherited a few things from him, especially the notion that she was just not good enough for anybody to want to be with. Well, his loss, she was beautiful now remember? She had been transformed. If only he could see her now!

But what was she thinking? How could she be different now? How could she look so wonderful?

She picked up the oval mirror and lifted it up. But there she was just like before, beautiful, like a painting, beauty that came from every angle and from the inside out. Her eyes glossy and filled with new life. She smiled a huge grin and put it down before going in to the bedroom and starting work on the wardrobe mirror. Trying, once more, not to look at herself in the reflection she unscrewed the glass and took it off the door disposing of it behind the wardrobe itself, never to be looked at again. If she never looked in another mirror she could fool herself that she was beautiful. If she only looked at herself in that dusty old antique she would look forever as she wished to look.

The new mirror was to take pride of place in the lounge and once it was hung she stood back and took a good look at herself. Could it really be her? Had she somehow had her prayers answered? Perhaps it was just that the mirror was dirty, a haze on the glass obscuring the truth. She promised herself that she would never clean it.

Hours later and Mona was still looking in the mirror. She could not get enough of the new her. She felt wonderful, confident, a different person entirely. In fact, she decided, she would go out with the girls. She could do it, she could be seen. She hadn't been out for so long she did not know if she would fit in to any of her dresses, but she didn't look fat now did she? She turned from side to side looking at her body in the reflection, and it was almost as if it belonged to someone else. She did not recognise the curves of this body. She undressed and looked at herself again, now naked, staring at every part, staring at the whole picture. Could it be true? She was sexy! Not skinny, for that would have been impossible, but her curves were voluptuous not fat. Her breasts were large and did not hang too low. Her belly was slight and did not stick out. She was a real woman, a beautiful woman. She could hardly contain her excitement.

Mona jumped up and down and screamed in delight trotting over to her stereo and putting it on, turning the volume up loud as the music began. And with the music filling her head she ran around the room, naked, happy, jumping and running and catching sight of herself in the mirror at every pass. She sang along to the songs, pretending to have a microphone in her hand, watching herself pose in front of the oval mirror.

Another hour slipped past and the CD had come to an end. Mona gave the reflection of herself a kiss and then skipped into the bedroom to get some dresses and dragged them all in to the lounge so that she could look in her new mirror as she tried them on. She looked fantastic in the black velvet, she looked fabulous in the red satin, she looked utterly gorgeous in the light blue cotton. Was there nothing that she could not wear? Every dress seemed to fit wonderfully around her frame. Nothing was too tight or too lose. She was spoilt for choices as to what she could wear that night.

It was nine o'clock and she had not decided. The girls were meeting at seven. But Mona was too infatuated to care about time. They were all used to her being late anyway. Another CD on the stereo, a few more dresses, a little more flirting with herself. They would miss her though wouldn't they? They had all wanted her to come. She would be the life and soul of the party wouldn't she? With her slender figure, her pouting red lips and deep brown eyes. They would be there right now all waiting for her.

She imagined it all. The moment of her entrance. Mouths would drop open and eyes would burn into her warming a red carpet along which she would walk. She would be wearing a long black dress that clung to her curvaceous body and every movement she made would be watched closely by her friends and the rest of the bar. And she would reach the bar itself and the bar tender would come straight over.

"What will it be?"

"Your best red wine, leave the bottle."

"I'll pay for that," a man would say at her side. A handsome man, dark haired with crystal blue eyes. "What's your name?"

And she could be anyone now couldn't she? A new life, a new persona.

"Marilyn." She would answer.

"You are the most divine woman I have ever seen."

And he would be the very model of everything she loved. His look would be strong yet gentle. His life in his eyes. Everything her ex was not. A man that knew the feelings of a woman yet was no less a man. A man that had a deep darkness that was infectious and beautiful.

He would be gone for a few minutes and the girls would surround her.

"He's gorgeous, you and he look great together."

"What do you think of him? If you don't want him I will. But he looks like he only has eyes for you Mona."

"Marilyn." Mona would say. A new name, a new life.

"You look so wonderful tonight."

And then they would be together declaring their love as if they had never experienced any time a part. And they could not suffer a moment longer that they would not be like this. Both of their lives meeting on this day as they always should. And she would marry him as soon as they could book the time. She would wear red and he would wear black trimmed in gold embroidery. They would look like angels. She would look as though she had fallen from heaven to make that ever lasting commitment. And their love would be that way forever because they both loved each other with equal devotion.

"No one is ever going to hurt you again."

Hours later and Mona found herself in her lounge, her head against the mirror a smile on her pretty mouth.

"Mona didn't turn up then."

It was eleven o'clock and the girls were drinking their last drinks before the bar shut up for the night.

"Probably for the best, she would only have made the rest of us look bad."

"I know. I might have not met Brian here if that one was loose amongst us!"

She tightened her grip around the man at her side.

"Mona is so gorgeous and such a nice person. Makes you kind of sick don't it?"

"Would have been nice to see her out of work though."

"Yeah, in some gorgeous dress made up to the nines."

"Well, we'll see her at work then I guess."

A Moment Gone

But Mona never did go back to work. Mona never left her living room. Mona never left her old oval mirror.

The Last Unicorn

When the last ray of hope dwindled into despair, when kindness became myth, the last unicorn died. No longer did that wild beauty roam the woods and glens of the pretty little village. Nature was robbed and nature was in sorrow. And years went by.

The hunt ran onwards, all red jackets and brown snorting horses. White hounds sniffing the ground as they ran ahead; tens of dogs with their lips rolled back to reveal their cruel teeth. The sound of the bugle and a ginger fox leapt from the under growth and sprang forward. Its speed was great but so was that of the horses, so were the hounds. The chase had begun.

The fox had heard tales of this happening in the old days, but never had he seen such a fearsome sight. His heart beat in his mouth and his breath was cold yet burnt in his throat. His legs seemed to be working without instruction, faster than they had ever worked before. It was life or death. Never had death been so close, never had he seen the reaper riding the horse in pursuit of he, the chosen. Never had life seemed so vital.

It went on, time meaning nothing, nothing meaning anything. But life was important, survival was the only thought. The fox ran on with the hounds so close, and that one horse with its great hooves thumping on the ground mere seconds behind him. He was sure to be caught, to be ripped apart, to be killed here, on this day. But then he

A Moment Gone

saw to his right a small clearing in the brush and he turned and jumped through it.

There was a moment of silence. The thundering noise of the horses, and the sniffling of the hounds was somewhere far away. Yet he did not stop, he ran on, leaping over fallen trees and diving under branches. He had time for another small thought... he might just survive this.

But he had run as far as he could go, he had reached a fast flowing stream that splashed white water over the sunken rocks. He had stopped, his heart pounding in his chest, his mouth burning with icy breath and there he stood, unable to move on, unable to hide. And that sound, like the beating of a great drum, the sound of horses was heard once more.

The little fox looked around him in the hope of a hiding place, but it was too late, a dark brown shape came closer and closer. Through the greenery he could see that it was a horse, yet his fear held off for there appeared to be no rider.

The horse slowed from a gallop to a trot and now came in to view past the last trees and into the clearing. The fox was quite sure that the horse was alone.

"Quick," the horse said, "jump up onto my neck and I will help you across the stream and run you to safety."

The fox was startled by the act of kindness but did not contemplate it for long. The sound of the hunter's horn came blowing through the bushes.

The fox jumped up on the horse and they were off, across the stream and then galloping along side it, out of the woods and across the fields, out and away. The horse made only a little conversation.

"The hunt is cruel," he said "and my master beats me. I have thrown him and now I will help you. I will live wild. Worry no more." And they were soon far away from the hunt and the hounds would no doubt have lost his scent completely. The fox was safe.

The horse eventually stopped where the stream grew wide and bent his neck to let the fox slide off onto the ground. It was only then that the fox saw the amazing transformation. The horse, once brown, had become a pure and startling white.

Look at yourself in the stream," he said in a gasp. And the horse looked.

"My." Said the horse. "I have changed haven't I?"

"It is magic. You look wonderful," the fox admired. "And thank you. I can not say thank you enough. You have saved my life and I owe you a debt. Thank you horse."

"You owe me no debt," the horse said, but the fox had stood up on his back legs and said:

"Let me pull away your muzzle." And as he said it he bit the leather around the horse's head and pulled him free. The horse could now begin its new life, wild and in peace. Then, again, the fox gasped in shock and said to the horse, "look again at yourself in the stream, you are changed still!"

And the horse looked and saw. There on the end of his great nose was a spiralling crystal white horn.

A Moment Gone

"It is a miracle," the fox said, "but you are a unicorn."

An act of kindness and once more nature smiled.

S. Westwood

And Another Suicide

It's easier for everyone if I do this thing today
Get it done
Get it over
Start to live again.

I'm guilty of the crime of selfish failure
To my mum
To my lover
Family and friends.

He is in me and his voice is always loud
The other me
The evil me
The dark and twisted suicide junkie.

I cannot fight him anymore
He made this decision for me
I love you
I'll miss you
And please know that I am sorry.

A Moment Gone

The Stars Become You

She would stand outside in the cold for hours just to look at the stars. Looking up to that vast expanse of navy darkness to see those specs of light burning furiously millions of miles into space. It can make you feel so small, so unimportant, yet at the same time part of something great. Nature, the world, and all of its natural beauties.

She would lose all sense of anything. She would lose herself, and he could never reach her.

"That's Orion," David said from behind her, an ignored finger pointing at one bright white star amidst the smaller twinkles. "At least, I think it is," he went on with an excusing tone, "I was looking it up the other day, on the internet." He was going to say more but she was not listening. It seemed that she never heard anything he said, so how would she ever know him? How could she ever love him?

"What?" She asked after minutes of silence had already past between them. She turned to face him for a moment, having asked what it was that he had said, but he knew she would not listen to his reply. He tried so hard to get through to her, but he could only ever get so far.

He slipped his arms around her waist to hold her close, feeling that he was with her for but a second, and then she was away. She was always so far away...

A little high pitched sound had caught her attention and she was searching in the darkness for the cat that had made such a pitiful noise.

"Come on," she called to it, crouching by the

bushes. And there it came, slow and timid, yet with an air of grace about its steps. An exquisite looking grey tabby cat with equal portions of sweetness and regal charm. It annoyed him. Damn cat, taking her attention. Damn stars. How could he compete?

Her affair with nature was a constant emotional torture. At least his only mistress was the inanimate, cream coloured set of boxes upon his desk: His computer.

He would spend hours searching the internet, finding things out that might give him some way to reach her. Talking to people that heard his typed out words and replied to him, giving their help. But it was only she that he loved. He had fallen in love with everything that was her, and although he wanted things to change, he would not change her for the world.

What was the answer? Computer, what is the answer?

The answer to her spirituality had a spiritual answer. It seemed that the forces of the nature she so loved could be manipulated in his favour. This he read, occasionally taking an excited yet nervous glance away from the screen and back to her. But she was not looking at all that he was reading; she was wistfully staring at one pure white fish as it gently glided through the clear aquarium water. She had no idea of the knowledge he was dissolving, the key he had been searching for every night for the last two years. From clue to clue, following one web site to another, until… the answer there, printing slowly onto paper, and then his forever.

A Moment Gone

She was out the next day, Sunday, the day she always went for a walk. He was alone and he had been to the supermarket, collecting all that he needed and checking it off his list. He had it all, he had mixed it as it told him he should, and he had those words printed on paper that he should read, read slowly, and make his magic work.

The web site had said that the spell came from an old Native American tradition. A ritual 'to bring man closer to nature, and bring nature to the man'.

So what if he had never believed in such things before? It had become the only answer. This was his chance, his only chance. He was not stupid, he could read between the lines and he knew what it was all about. He had heard tales of shape changing and of man becoming a beast. He knew what it all could mean. He was even clever enough to change some of the ingredients to suit the modern age. And he was clever enough to sacrifice the neighbor's cat in exchange for 'wolf's blood'. That was where he had really excelled himself, cutting its throat and adding the cat's blood to the mixture in the cup.

If there was some truth to it all, then she would love him, and he would have her love. If it did not work then at least he would know that he had tried his best. He had done everything in his power. He had followed the instructions. He had drunk that potion and read those words. Now he just had to wait...

She came home at four as usual, and with a breezy air of refreshed senses she hung her coat upon its hook and walked into the living room.

There she stopped dead in her tracks.
"David?"

The room was a mess. A circle had been made with candles, now burnt down to stubs, paper was thrown about the floor, and a cup of something had been spilt on the carpet staining it black, or, it seemed, burning straight through it. Amongst all this was David, lying on his stomach, eyes rolled back in his head and mouth slack and blue.

"David?"

But it was no use. David was dead now: Man brought closer to nature, and nature brought to the man.

A Moment Gone

New York Punk

They should have realised that something was wrong when I stopped listening to the Ramones and began listening to the Smiths. The Ramones just suddenly seemed too damn happy - I could empathise much more with Morrissey and his lyrics 'Heaven knows I'm miserable now'. But my family had no idea.

No matter how many times I staggered down the stairs with an empty bottle of cheap cider to put in the dustbin, they were happily oblivious. No matter how loudly I played that song 'asleep', with those lines... 'I would be so glad to go' my parents remained completely in the dark about my change of mind. What would it take to make them sit up and notice?

It took fifty paracetamol and a broken bic disposable razor.

I knew that I would probably not die. I had not taken enough pills and all the slashes on my arms were superficial, but while I held the blade between my fingers and drew the blood from my own skin- I knew that I would be happy with whatever result occurred. Let me die- Let me get help- Let me be scarred like a tattoo displaying my anguish. I did not care; I only wanted something to change- just like my music taste.

My mother found me in the morning, incoherent and covered in crusted blood. She called the ambulance, and before I knew it I had become part of the mental health system. I was visited by social workers- I was talked at by psychiatrists. I was given pills to increase those joyful chemicals they said my brain was lacking, and my family were all concerned.

But what had all this achieved? Now everyone knew, and now everyone cared. I had become this fragile creature to watch over and wrap in cotton wool. I was checked up on and made to answer the telephone- just because people would presume I was dead if I failed to answer the damn thing!

Maybe if I could just play a little New York punk, things will go back to normal.

A Moment Gone

The Story of the Snugglewumps

For my little boy, Draven Saul x

"My mum said that the wood was not there when she was really little."

"That's rubbish," Martin said with a hint of annoyance in his voice. "Trees grow real slow you know. Them trees have been there for years and years. They don't even have leaves anymore, that means they're dead and only old things die."

Tom believed what his mum had said because he never doubted what his parents told him, but he had to admit that he did not think trees really grew as fast as that. The trees in the wood were huge. Some of them had trunks so big that he and Martin could stand holding hands, trying to hug the tree all the way round but only getting half way round. Years of growth would be needed to make a tree that big. He had learnt at school how if you chopped down a tree you could count the circles printed on the inside of the trunk to see how old it had been. Each circle was a year. Some of the trees were so big that he guessed they had been growing there for hundreds of years. He thought about it a while, thinking of how those trees had stood watching the world go by. How many children had climbed their branches, and how many people had they seen grow up? How his own mother could have played in the leaves that fell from it in autumn all those years ago, before they had all died. The wood must have been there.

"Ok," Tom said, "Let's plant a tree and see

how long it takes."

"Ok," Martin answered laughing a little, "but don't expect it to be exciting! You'll see I'm right."

The next day was warm and sunny and nature had woken early to enjoy the day. Lying in his bed, Tom listened to the tens of bird songs and watched the few clouds drifting by from his window. He cuddled his favourite teddy bear, 'wump' a name that stuck because the bear had a hump on his back and when he was younger he could not pronounce his h's. It was his parents that called it his 'snuggle wump' as he always had it close and snuggled. It was a lovely long haired bear, soft and cuddly and had little fairy wings on its back. Tom was sure the bear was like him, gentle, quiet and, generally, good. It was a grown up bear and always looked after the other toys.

His friend Martin had a bear too, a multi coloured little thing that was probably supposed to be a friendly, hairy monster. But his bear was probably more like Martin was, mischievous and naughty. Tom called it a 'mugwump' but Martin, trying to be hard and grown up said it was 'just a bear'. He never said that when they were younger. When they were younger their 'wumps' had all sorts of adventures.

After a while Tom got up, remembering what he was planning to do.

His father had found him an old bag of compost and had told him where in their massive garden he could plant his tree. His family were very rich and he had a lovely garden to play in and a big house to get lost in. In fact, the whole village was full of big houses and happy people.

A Moment Gone

"Plant an apple tree," his dad said, "we could use an apple tree."

"Where do I get tree seeds?" Tom asked and his parents giggled a little and looked at each other. Then his mother went in the house for a moment before coming out with an apple in her hand. She threw it for Tom to catch, and he did catch it.

"Are you sure he should plant it *there*," his mother said, nudging his dad with her arm.

"He is only a child," his father said to his mum, a little sternly. Tom didn't understand why. "He should plant the tree in the garden so he can see how long it takes to bear fruit."

"But it will take years," his mother said.

Tom's dad seemed to be a little cross but it made no sense to him why.

"It's a lesson for him," his father said.

"Will it really take years?" Tom asked.

"In the garden it will," his mother said, still looking his father in the eyes and giggling to herself, a joke only she seemed to understand.

"Yes." His father said. "Trees take a long time to grow and even longer to bear fruit."

"And I just plant the apple?" Tom asked.

His mother began to laugh again.

"Eat the apple," his father said, "and deep inside you will find the core, the bit you don't eat, and there are little seeds in there. You plant them."

Tom stood looking down at the apple in his hand and then up to his parents. Something strange was going on between his mother and father but he was too young to understand it. He ate the apple, and sure enough, he found the little

S. Westwood

brown seeds. He had to wait a while for Martin to come round to his house and he had about five seeds laid out on a piece of kitchen towel waiting. Then they set to work.

They dug a small hole and filled it half way with compost, then they put the seeds in. They watered the seeds, half expecting some instant reaction, green shoots growing up from the little brown seeds. But nothing happened. They put the rest of the compost on and added a little more water, then stood back. Still nothing happened and although Tom had expected no different he was still a little disappointed. The two boys left the garden, and as usual they went to the wood.

"This wood is so dense and the trees are so big there's no way they weren't here when your mum was our age."

"Wel my mum said it so…"

"She's telling you porky pies." Martin said.

"You'll see." Tom answered.

The next day Tom went to the place where they had planted the tree to see if anything had happened. There was nothing. There was nothing the day after that, and the day after that and quite frankly, Tom was annoyed. He decided to ask his mother.

"Mum, my tree hasn't started to grow yet."

"It won't," she smiled and looked around her as if to check that no one was listening. "But the woods that you play in," she whispered, "are magic! They weren't there until we planted the trees there in spring and they grew and grew over a few weeks until they were as big as houses. Then they

A Moment Gone

blossomed. Then they bore their fruits and we picked them all right away. Then the leaves turned yellow and red and died. The trees bore no more fruit after that. So we planted more. We planted them all."

"So my tree wont grow?"

"Oh it will grow, but it will take years. If you really want to prove your friend wrong you have to plant your tree in the woods."

Tom had his mouth open, gasping at what he was being told and about to ask another question but then his father entered the room. His mum put a finger to her mouth, the signal that the conversation had been secret.

"What are you doing home in weather like this?" His father said. "Go make the most of the sun."

Tom ran out, but not before grabbing an apple from the fruit bowl.

Martin laughed when his friend explained to him about the woods.

"That's the stupidest thing I ever heard."

"You'll see."

Tom believed his mother and had already got the seeds from the apple. It wasn't long before they had reached the woods and Tom was digging a hole with his hands. He dropped the seeds in and pushed the soil back over the top. Then he waited.

"This is dumb." Martin laughed. Tom continued to stare at the patch of earth. He stood and he stared and he felt a breeze catch his brown hair and blow it into his eyes. He brushed his hair aside and there he saw, moving up through the black dirt, a fresh green shoot of a plant, or of a flower, or of his tree. Martin stopped laughing. There it was, growing upwards, dancing side to side to a silent song.

"Wow!" Martin exclaimed.

"Didn't I tell you?" Tom said, defiant. "My mum told me it will grow within days." And as they watched, it had already grown to the height of their knees and had already got green branches and green leaves. "But it will only live a year, that's the sad part."

"You can't feel sad about a tree." Martin scoffed.

"We will have to pick all the apples straight away is all."

"Why?"

"I'm not really sure... I think they'll go bad otherwise. So we pick them all straight away."

"Cool. Does your mum know anymore little secrets?"

"I don't think so. But my dad doesn't even want me to know this one."

Days did pass and everyday the boys went back to see how high and how wide the tree had grown. By the second day it had already grown as high as the two boys. By the third it was already strong enough to climb. It was a fully grown adult tree within just four days and that's when the white blossom came decorating the whole tree like snow.

"See, see! Next we'll get the apples."

Well the blossom fell and in its place grew little buds. Then the buds broke to reveal the tree's

A Moment Gone

fruits. But there were no bright green shinny apples. No round plump fruits to pick and eat. All there was were overgrown, brown and oval apple seeds.

"What the heck are they?" Martin said in his usual tactless taunt.

"I think," Tom said, "they are apple seeds."

"Apple seeds?"

Tom was thinking, rubbing his head and thinking so hard that he had blocked off the mocking of his friend, concentrating on trying to work out why this had happened and remembering conversations he had been having with his mother.

"They *are* apple seeds!" He said. "Because that's what we planted!"

"What?"

"If we plant an apple, then we'll get apples!"

Martin looked unconvinced.

"It's true... let's do it."

And so they did- that very day- they planted an apple just as if it were a seed, and again they stood by in awe as it grew before their eyes.

A few days later, in the height of summer the blossom had formed, and later the blossom fell and revealed luscious green apples.

"It's true!" Martin said, obviously surprised.

"Wow. We could grow anything." Tom said, thinking of all the fruits they could grow, thinking that they could sell them and make some good money.

"Yes. We could," Martin said, very excited. I'll go get something."

Twilight had started to fall by the time the boys met up again at the wood. They went passed the tree that they had first planted and noticed that all the large apple seeds had fallen to the ground and the leaves of the tree were already brown. There apple tree, however, was lush and ripe.

In amongst the trees it was already dark and the birds had stopped singing.

"What did you bring?" Tom asked.

Martin held out his hand, and there in his palm were three plastic army men.

"Why have you got them?" Tom asked.

"We can grow anything right? Then I want some more of these."

"I don't think that's going to work."

"Well I want to try."

So they did. They buried the little plastic men and they watched as the green shoot reached out of the dirt.

The wait to see the trees fruits was unbearable and, although Tom did not really think it would work, his mind was going crazy with possibilities.

"Wow… look!"

The tree had grown big and strong in the few days they had left it and in amongst its green leaves were hundreds of little plastic men.

"It worked!"

The boys were amazed, though perhaps not completely surprised. Why wouldn't it work? Tom's mum had practically told them the secret.

"Yes," Tom looked serious, "but we don't know the rules. What if we don't pick them all?"

"Well they can't die, they're just toys!" Martin laughed. "The first trees we planted have died already so I'll pick all the men now. I want to pick

A Moment Gone

them all. I want to play with them. Wow! What an army. We can have anything we want can't we. Hey! Your mum and dad know about this. Have you ever wondered why everyone in the village is rich? They've been planting money. That's what they've all done. They've planted money and the trees have grown it. Wow! We can have anything."

Tom began to wonder if he should have told his friend about this. He began to have a real bad feeling about it.

Well the two boys spent the rest of the day hitting the tree's branches with sticks catching all the fallen toys in a bucket. By the time the darkness fell the bucket was full and the tree was bear.

"I think we have them all." Martin said at length.

"Good." Tom said, exhausted, I thought it would never end.

Their eyes scanned each branch, looking for those little plastic men but by now their eyesight was blurring from hours of looking and the visibility was beginning to fade.

"What if we missed some?" Tom said, worried.

"So what? Look how many we have! You can have half and I'll have half. Tomorrow we'll plant something else. I can't wait!"

For some reason Tom was not as excited as his friend, he really did have a bad feeling about it all. He had always been taught that just because you want something it does not mean you can just have it. When he had wanted a new toy he had to wait for his birthday or for Christmas. There was a good feeling when he had saved enough of his pocket money to buy a new video game. He liked to be paid in sweets when he washed his dad's car. It just didn't seem right to be growing toys.

He did not see his friend Martin the next day at school, and he never called for him later that evening. Tom did not mind but obviously wondered why. Perhaps it was for the best. He thought to himself that as his friend did not come in to school for the next few days, a dose of the flu might make him forget all about growing trees.

It was at about midnight, four days since he had last seen Martin, when he heard a noise at his window. He woke with a start and sat up, scared at what it might be, scared of monsters and 'bad men'. His curtains began to move and he heard a strange human noise, a 'gruphing' sound. He pushed himself back against the wall, staring at the moving curtains. And as they parted he saw Martin, struggling in through the window and falling down onto his floor. As soon as Martin was in he composed himself, got up, and looked back out the window before quickly shutting the curtains and turning to his friend who was still shaken with previous fear.

"Mate," He said. "I've got a problem."

"What is it?" Tom said rubbing his sleepy eyes and sitting up straighter in the bed.

"Mugwumps." Martin said, a serious, tired expression on his face.

"What?!" Tom didn't understand.

"If you don't pick them, they come alive."

"What do? Pick what?" If Tom wasn't so

A Moment Gone

sleepy he might have made more sense of his friend's plight but in the middle of the night it just sounded daft.

"I planted my toy, you know, the mugwump? In the woods. It grew like the army men. There were lots of them, mugwumps on every branch." Martin was staring at his friend with huge eyes, but stopped for a second to look through the curtains again before turning back. "I think I've shaken them off."

"You mean the mugwumps came alive?"

"The ones I didn't pick yes."

"Which was how many?"

"Well I haven't been well... I couldn't get back to the wood."

"Which is how many?"

"Kind of... well, all of them."

"So there are hundreds of little mugwumps running around?"

"Yes."

"What are they like?"

"Well they're kind of... naughty."

"Naughty?"

"Yes.

They trampled the flowers in my garden. I got told to stay in my room and think about what I had done. Then they got in to my room and ripped all my posters. They tore my favourite 'Harry Potter' one and everything. Then they made a right mess, my toys were everywhere."

"What did your parents say?"

"Well as soon as my parents came in the room to see what all the noise was about they all hid under the bed. They saw the mess and grounded me. I had to wait till night to come here and they were all following me."

"What if they get in here?"

Martin looked through the curtains again.

"I think I lost them."

"Well what do we do?"

"Couldn't you ask your mum? She knows about the woods doesn't she?"

"My dad will be cross if he finds out."

"So what else can we do?"

Tom thought. He thought so much that his brain began to hurt. All he could think of was to get someone to take the mugwumps in hand. To teach them not to be naughty. To tell them that they are grounded or send them to their rooms to think about how naughty they had been. They needed about fifty mummy's to tell each one of them off. And as he thought he looked down at his bear, his own wump, his snugglewump, the toy that had always been good to him through his childhood and a toy he could not imagine would ever be naughty.

"You always get me into trouble" Tom said.

"Yeah and you always sort it out."

"Yes, well I do have an idea." He said and held his bear up to his friend. "We teach those mugwumps how to behave!"

The next morning was a Saturday. Just as well because they were going to be busy. Martin had spent all night on Tom's floor and left before anyone else had woken up. He went home as quickly as he could through the devastation that was once a quiet neighbourhood. There were bent lampposts, bins on the floor with their contents

A Moment Gone

thrown about, a crashed, abandoned car, and out the corner of his eye he could see things, little colourful things, darting behind trees and under parked cars, and a high pitched giggling from all directions. Oh dear. The mugwumps had been busy making a mess all night. But they were good at hiding. Martin knew they were all regrouping, he could hear them, as he walked they followed. He had to lead them away from the town before they were seen; before questions were asked and he gets in trouble. Thank God he had a friend in Tom.

Back at his house Martin climbed the tree beside his window and climbed in. He had played that trick so many times, all those times he had been grounded and he hated missing out on fun. He looked down into the garden and there he saw them, all the little mugwumps, those colourful little monster bears with their big clumsy feet, climbing up the tree. He closed his window, then his curtains, and then he made his way out of his bedroom to begin the façade of normality.

Tom hoped his idea would work. The town was in chaos. He pretended to know nothing about it when his parents discussed the mayhem that was going on outside. Like some invisible riot. Sightings of little creatures that the news broadcast put down to mass hysteria. But Tom knew all too well what was happening. He had to help. But his parents said, given the circumstances, he should not be allowed to go out. What was he to do?

He went to his room and sat on his bed thinking about what a mess had been caused and blaming himself. He should never have confided in Martin. He wondered if he should tell his mum the truth.

Just then he heard a noise at his window. He looked quickly around and stared at the glass worried as to what caused the tap sound. The noise came again and he saw it came from a small stone. Were the mugwumps throwing stones at his window? He hardly dared to look out. Another stone hit the glass and Tom looked. There was his friend Martin, standing in the garden below, a mugwump sitting on his head, ruffling up his hair.

Tom opened his window.

"Come on we have to do something quick." Martin called up.

"I can't. My mum won't let me out."

"What was your plan?"

Tom thought for a moment about his plan and about whether it would work. He looked to his bed and to his snugglewump that sat on the pillow.

At the window Tom called to his friend.

"Take this and plant it," he called holding the snugglewump out of the window. He let it drop and Martin went to pick it up off the lawn. "Don't pick them when they grow. Then they'll come alive and sort out your mess."

"How?"

"Just trust me."

"Well it better work."

"Well if it doesn't you can always plant your army men again!"

"I don't want to hurt the little things." Martin said finally shaking off the mugwump in his hair. The little monster bear ran off into the flower bed and started trampling the flowers.

"You better be quick." Tom said.

A Moment Gone

There was a knock at Tom's bedroom door and then it opened. His mother came in with a serious look on her face.

"Tom," she started. "Can you tell me the truth about something."

Tom knew what was coming. Over the last few days there had been numerous sightings of little colourful, fluffy creatures and everyone's gardens were a mess. The news was reporting daily about more havoc taking place in their little town. No one was getting hurt but lots of annoying things were happening to resident's property. TV aerials were being bent, signposts were pointing the wrong way, there were strange muddy foot prints on people's cars, and someone, or something, had put washing up liquid in the fountain causing white bubbles that spread all over the park. His mum knew something.

"Did you plant something in the woods?" she asked sternly.

Tom did not know if he should come clean or cover for his friend. Then he thought that he would rather have his mum's help and off loading his secret would be easier than a web of lies.

"Martin planted his toy. His mugwump. And he forgot to pick them when they grew. But I am sorting it out. I'm going to plant my snugglewump."

"Will that make it better?" his mum asked.

"I think so... I have a plan but I need to go out."

"Well, you better go out and help your friend. Water the tree and it will grow quicker. You need to sort this mess out don't you?" She sounded a little sharp, as if se were disappointed in him yet there was a sparkle in her eyes that seemed to convey something else.

"Sorry mummy," he said.

"Magic needs respect," his mother said, that sparkle lighting up her face, "and you have to be careful with knowledge. Go now, water the tree and help your friend."

Tom saw more of the mess he had caused on his way to the woods. Bent lampposts, traffic lights stuck on red, and, and as he walked down the street he noticed that all the house numbers had been moved about. 1,4,7,2... The mugwumps had changed them all around. Oh dear, this was a shambles. He blamed himself. He called for Martin on his way and his friend answered the door looking very disheveled.

"Oh Tom. I did it, I planted the bear."

"Not a bear," Tom said, "a snugglewump. Remember how we used to play with them?"

"Yes I remember. I also remember all the things I made my mugwump do. I remember how he broke your toys."

"Mmmm," Tom remembered. "We need to water the tree to make it grow quicker."

"Will that make a difference?"

"Yes. Well my mum said watering it would make it grow quicker. We'll try it." And Tom had brought a watering can with him, filled with water that was proving rather heavy. "Lets go."

In the woods they rushed to the snugglewump tree and there they saw the little tree with small buds on every branch. Tom poured the water at the base of the trunk and they watched as the tree grew bigger as they watched and the buds

A Moment Gone

blossomed in to winged little bears hanging from every branch, their backs humped and their hair shaggy. If they picked them they would just be toys. If they let them drop off like leaves in autumn they would come alive. That was the plan.

Tom did not know if watering the tree again would make any difference now that the tree had grown but he did it anyway. He poured the water around the base of the tree and then both boys stood back to watch.

For a few minutes nothing happened but then it began. One of the bears began to fall and when it was close to landing on the floor its orange gossamer wings began to flap really fast and the bear flew up and flew up, hovering around the tree looking at the boys. Then another fell, and another and each one flapped its wings and became animated before they landed, they came alive. The snugglewumps were all alive! Now they were all flapping their wings as fast as a bee waiting, it seemed, for the boys to say something.

"Listen snugglewumps!" Tom called. "The mugwumps are naughty and need to be looked after. Please help!"

The bears all looked at one another and then looked back to Tom and nodded. They all flew off in the direction of the town. Now they could only hope that Tom's idea would work. The boys left the woods, just catching sight of the little bear swarm fading in to the distance.

The boys sat on the swings in the park for a while. Of course they had to get the knots out of the swing's chains first for the mugwumps had been there at some point and left their mark. But as the boys sat there swinging they did not see any sign of the colourful little wumps. They sat and they talked about what their parents' had said about the mess in town.

"My father said that he had seen stranger things," Martin said.

"And my mother knew what we had done," Tom said.

"How did she know?" Martin asked, concerned.

"You know... they just know. My mum always knows if I'm lying or hiding something. She knew we had planted something."

"Then they must have done something like this themselves."

"Possibly."

The town was quiet as they walked back to their homes. They walked past all the shops, past parked cars with muddy hand prints on their windows. They walked through the mess that was left from every litter bin that the mugwumps had emptied. They arrived back home without seeing a single wump of either type and could only hope that Tom's plan had worked. They got to Tom's house they saw Martin's family car parked outside.

"Hello boys." Martin's dad called out as they came in to the house. Their parents were all sitting in the lounge drinking tea.

"We've been talking about you." Martin's mum said as the boys stood in the doorway.

"We're all going for a little walk."

Tom and Martin looked at one another. Any

A Moment Gone

minute the sparks would fly. Any minute now their parents were going to give them a right telling off.

"Where are we going?" Martin asked as they began their walk.

"To the woods." His dad answered. "Do you know, there was no wood at all when we were your age. We planted the whole lot."

They knew, they all knew.

But it was getting dark. The boys were never allowed out this late and they certainly did not like the idea of being in the woods when it was dark.

The walk seemed to last forever. A silence had fallen over them and it was very uncomfortable. The woods were not far though and just before they got there their parents stopped, signaling the others to stop too. They stood and looked ahead to the trees, little flickering lights dancing amongst the dead branches.

"What's that?" Martin asked in a gasp.

"Let's go see," his mother answered.

They went tentatively in, finding a big enough gap between two trees where the undergrowth was not so thick. Inside there was a world of wonder. The snugglewumps were flying around and the mugwumps were all there too, sitting in a circle around a little fire in the middle. One of the snugglewumps was in the middle too talking to the assembled group. There were little candles handing from tree branches lighting up the whole wood. None of the creatures paid any notice to the humans that had walked in to the wood. But what an amazing sight! It seemed like the snugglewumps were teaching the mugwumps as if they were at school- teaching them how to behave no doubt, just as Tom had planned!

"You sorted it out very well," Tom's mum said, "And I guess I should blame myself. We planted all sorts when we were younger. The trick is to pick them before they fall. Still no real harm done. Accept the mess in town... now who's going to clean that?" To the boys's surprise she was not cross. And in the few seconds that she had the boy's attention there was no hint of anger.

"Well," Martin said, "if we planted some toy dustmen..."

A Moment Gone

Sorry

They said that I should count myself lucky that I was lying in a hospital bed rather than the hospital morgue, but I did not feel lucky. When you attempt suicide you expect to die not to have to deal with even more than there was before you took the pills. Now I had to witness the affect my potential death was having on everyone, especially my mother whose reactions constantly changed from grief to anger and then to total bewilderment.

"Why?" She kept on saying. And then she would repeat things that seemed so trivial that my mind would filter them out before giving them any thought. "You're loved, you're young and handsome…Why Adam?"

I just lay there, on my back, looking ahead at the orange curtains drawn around the bed, the pattern on them dancing slowly, pulsing. The pills were making me hallucinate, but there was no pleasure in it. I felt like those optical illusions would never end, that my brain had been, somehow, permanently damaged. The patterns were faces of demons, grimacing gargoyles that would not stop moving.

I closed my eyes. There was an empty feeling in my guts, as if the pills had burnt me away inside. Little needle-like pains were sparking my nerves every now and again, and there was a tingling sensation in the tips of my fingers. I felt broken, I felt sick, and I felt truly afraid to still be alive.

No, I did not count myself lucky.

Sooner or later the psychiatrists would come

and try to find out why I did it, whether I was crazy, and if I was likely to try it again. But they would get nothing out of me. They cannot read minds, they only know from you what you let them know, and I would think before I spoke. I would tell them what they needed to hear in order to be let out. No one would ever understand that I had no choice, that it was the only feasible option.

My mind was going crazy, as it had for so many years, but I had to concentrate on acting normal, pretending that I felt sorry for what I had done, rather than just sorry that it had not worked. It was a moment of weakness, I would have them believe, and I was now ok and ready to go back home. But in actual fact I was scared to go back home. In actual fact, being alive at all was scaring me to death! How was I supposed to move on from this? The only answer I could find was that I would have to try it again.

It seemed like my mother would never leave; in fact I began to worry that she may never leave me alone again. How the hell was I supposed to get out of this world if she was going to be watching me like a shadow? She still sat there on that cushioned chair to the left of the bed, leaning forward with her clasped hands held up to rest her chin. I saw how her fingers would keep clenching nervously, her red painted nails digging into her own skin. She did not even look directly at me, as if she could not bear to. I was her son, come from her body, and trying to leave my own. Two steps from death with my hand plugged into a drip, speaking no words, but thinking plenty.

She was not speaking either by then;

A Moment Gone

perhaps she had run out of new ways to say the same thing. Give her time and she would think of something else and start again, blasting me with the guilt as to how selfish I had been to not consider the family's feelings. But guilt was no stranger to me, in fact, guilt was just one of the many reasons why suicide had become my welcome friend.

I prayed for death, I crossed my fingers in hopeless hope. But there I lay, my body getting slowly healthier while my mind died through its endless torture.

"I'm sorry."

Sorry I could never get my mother to see inside my head. Sorry that I could not tell anyone my feelings. Sorry I had to live.

A/S/L

He sits at the screen again, legs straddling the rickety swivel chair that seems to wince at his ample weight. He has never had the time to replace it. His fingers tap straight onto the keys he knows so well, the password that he types without even seeing it as a word anymore, just a rhythm of fingertips on plastic keys. And the image blinks, the computer crunches, and his world opens.

This has been his universe for months, the computer a replacement for the woman who walked out as the delivery man walked in, parcel carried into the lounge.

He is not even awake yet; he has no time to wait for that privilege. The world will not wait, the text will change if you blink, the website will update if you turn your back. Maybe someone had added a comment; maybe someone would e-mail him as he read that comment. It will not end, back and forth, never missing a thing.

His hand reaches for the mug of coffee he had quickly made while the connection was finalizing - one eye looking round the door at the monitor. He was lucky this time; he made it in time. It tastes good, smooth, comforting. Every comfort he needs is here now.

So what that he is not dressed. So what if his hair looks terrible and unwashed, and his face is covered with stubble? No one can see him. There are people in there, others like him, looking into their screens across the miles, down the cables and into his home.

'Anyone wanna chat with female, 22, UK?'

A Moment Gone

'Yes' he types quickly before he is beaten too it, 'I am male, 24, UK'

His photograph is on the top right of the screen. He looks good in that picture, young and fresh. Yes, he had looked that good once, all those years ago when he really was only 24. But he could be whatever age he wanted could he not? Who was he hurting? This was his world, and who would ever know that he was not all those things he ever wished he was? A fifty-year-old man has to find his comforts somewhere.

S. Westwood

I only like your eyes because I can see me
reflected in them
I only like your soul because it reminds me of me
I only like your mind because it makes mine
superior

And what else is left of you?
You live and it is ugly
Life is ugly
But what of me?
I'm as ugly as life.

A Moment Gone

Call of the Sea

She said that the waves sang to her, but I could never hear their song. Just a lot of rushing whispers breaking before you catch their meaning. But she would stand there for hours, feet rooted in the pebbles, mind dancing on the surf. No one ahead of her for hundreds of miles, everything behind; that is what she told me, that was her fascination. And what did I understand of it? What did I understand of her? A country boy- brought up with the trees, sleeping in leaves and sniffing in the healthy decay of nature's regeneration. The sea was a mystery to me.

"The sea is a mystery, that is the point." She had said.

It scared me, that is my honesty. It scared me how much she could be lost to it, and lost to me. And the sea itself, endless and powerfully unstoppable, that was a fear that had a name.

We were married, and the sea was her affair. We would argue, and that was where she would always go. We would have problems; things that needed solving, things that needed talking through, but she would leave me in order to stand by herself on that barren beach.

If I tried real hard, I could see her from our window. I could crane my neck and squint my eyes to see her there, completely still but for her dark hair as it caught on the breezes. And, eventually, she would come home.

"She says that you should take the job."
"The sea? The sea tells you this?"
"It is what she thinks is right."

And was it ever wrong? The new job made me happy; it made us both happy. The money was good, and we made wonderful friends from the people I worked with.

"Don't worry baby, everything's going to be ok."

"You don't know that Amy…How can you know that?"

"I know…"

And somehow things always were. The problems of one day were forgotten the next, like the memory of a harsh winter, lost in the comforting heat of summer.

"Tonight honey…" She said dreamily.

"Tonight what Amy?"

"Tonight we make love and tonight I love you as if this was our last night on Earth."

She was gone when I woke; I did not have to guess where. And I hung out of my window like I had so many times before, straining my eyes over the roof tops to see her there.

She walked towards the sea; I saw it clear enough. And the water lapped at her feet and kissed her ankles. The waves bowed to her and hugged her legs for a while. Yet even from that distance I could see what was happening. As the sea dragged back from her body, taking leave to renew itself, I could see how her legs had changed. Her naked, slender legs were now no longer legs at all. She belonged to the sea now, as surely as any creature that lived within its depths. And I had to let her go, for she had given herself to it. Amy, my beautiful girl, now the sea's own mermaid with her

A Moment Gone

silver tail glinting in the white early morning sun. My beautiful Amy, riding each new wave further and further away from me.

And now I had some little understanding, just as somehow I knew that the sea would be the end of us, and I knew that I could never compete.

As I grew old, the sea was immortally fresh. As I became stagnant, the sea was always changing. As I would slowly lose my wits, the sea is forever wise. And as I hold onto nothing, the sea keeps it safe.

Obsession

If he had a pound for every heartbreak, he would have three pounds fifty: A pound for Sarah, one for Michelle and one for Amber. He was still with Beth, yet it broke his heart a little more each day. He loved her so much that every other breath he gave to her; every other heartbeat was hers and one part of his brain was dedicated to constant thoughts of her. It was no way to live; it was a half-life, yet he could not give it up. What did money matter anyway? What did anything matter but her? He would rather give her his entire being than be without her. What had he even been without Beth in his life?

Once there had been a boy, his name had been David, and it still was, but he was not that boy any longer. That boy would smile and drink, sleep and eat. He did none of these pointless things anymore. Beth was fuel for his body; he had starved before he met her. He had tried to survive on a minuscule diet of Sarah, Michelle and Amber. He had tried to lead a life always in the knowledge that he was waiting for it to really begin.

She loved him, and it was so unlikely that when she spoke the words the air filled with poison gasses that tightened the arteries around his heart. When she held him in her arms he shrank away, lost between them, and becoming nothing. Being with her was as cruel as being away. Being away was like being severed from his umbilical cord while hanging over some great chasm. Yet being with her was like being within the womb, knowing that it was only a matter of time before he was pushed

A Moment Gone

out.

How could he have let himself get like this? How did he become so dependant on something so out of control?

He wished he had four pounds, that fifty pence more: Just enough to buy the pills that would heal his heart ache forever.

S. Westwood

When They Came, And They Stole The World

There was a time when such things were mere folk tales, a time when those folk tales once had an ounce of truth and a time when they all came true.

I was fifteen when it started, life was just beginning, yet how was I to know? How could anyone guess at such strange things? Fairy folk were the wistful tales told to children at bedtime. They were the sweet, innocent creatures in beautiful ethereal pictures. They were glorious dreams of pretty girls with sparkling, diaphanous wings. They were a danger to no one, not even in your wildest imaginings. They were myths. They were something to wish for, to hope for, to secretly come to collect your fallen teeth and replace them with a bright shinning coin under your pillow. How were we to know?

But such things, it has since been said, have always existed. Even before the human beings, so dominant on this world for so long, they have been. Ever since Eve's first children were banished by God himself, to be unseen forever, they had been, and they had been plotting.

We stole our time on Earth, the human beings, all thinking there were no threats to us but ourselves. We sat back and were complacent. We were fools; but happiness comes more freely to the ignorant. I would give anything to still believe that those things were merely something to believe in, but never to see. I so wish I had never seen it, but at least I was a young man by then, at least I had been safe...

A Moment Gone

They came at night. There was no forewarning. They came when darkness covered our sight and sleep shrouded our minds. Those of us who had babies, and those of us who had children no older than three years of age, were all visited during those long dark hours. Some of us woke intuitively, or perhaps it was that sound of distant commotion, but we woke to find our windows and doors all wide open, the breeze whipping in and through our rooms, entering our houses and stealing our young.

Something had taken my baby brother Jacob from his cot. He had only been one year old. Nothing there now but the blue knitted blankets thrown aside and the indent of his small body on the white sheets.

Something had taken Mary, the sweet little girl next door with her white blonde hair and crystal blue eyes.

Something had taken the children. Something had taken them all.

As the light of dawn brought further realisations to our town, the sound of the mother's crying was deafening. No sound had ever been so pitiful, it filled the streets and it echoed through our homes. Nothing had ever happened that was anymore devastating than this. And no one knew. No one had any idea what had happened.

The televisions and radios were full of no other news but this. For it was not isolated to our town, the very same thing had happened throughout the entire country. And as each country in the world had its night, each one had its very own disaster. It happened everywhere, and all the children were gone.

As the news broadcasts continued the whole story slowly unfolded. There had been sightings, and although ignored at first, each one bared too much resemblance to the next to be seen as anything less than proof. People had seen little creatures, one foot tall at the most, creatures with protruding lips and long, thick matted hair. People had seen these things dragging sacks behind them, sacks containing our children, and they had seen their wings unfold behind them as they took flight away from sight. But the sightings were quick, those creatures were too fast, and those creatures were fairies.

I am nearing forty years old, and all this happened twenty-five years ago, yet it is as clear in my mind now as it was back then. My memory is refreshed at least once a year by the fact that this happens again and again. If a neighbor has a child, I am waiting in fear for the morning to come, and for their sobs to fill my ears. Nothing that the governments, the police or the people do to prevent it seems to mean a thing.

We are no nearer to uncovering their secrets. We know neither from where they come nor to where they go. We do not know where are babies have gone, or whether they still live. We have tried every way to shut them out, yet still they come, and still they steal. There are never any children, not for long, and people have given up on conceiving. There is little point in anything and no hope to wish for.

These are dark times, and these are the last times the human race will ever know.

A Moment Gone

The Artist

"It's wonderful, you're quite the artist."

"You flatter me Lucy."

"No, really," Lucy said moving a hand through her red hair with unintentional flirtation. Her dark eyes looked up at him, and then back down to the masterpiece she found herself admiring so much. "The trees, they are exquisitely abstract; so perfect yet without perfection. There is no symmetry to any of this, yet it seems so right."

"There is symmetry," he said as though hurt, defending his work. "You see the petals of this flower, they are equal sizes all around it."

"Well, not really," Lucy explained delicately, and pointed to one of the red petals. "You see, if you look closely, that one there is raised slightly higher than the others...but it isn't a criticism, it is what makes it so personal."

"Well, what do you make of my people-have they not got perfection?"

"He looks like you, and she me."

"Then I have achieved what I meant to. And do they not have symmetry?"

"They do, I agree. The eyes are equal, and his magnificently blue, like yours, like the seas, like the skies. Hers you have made green, as are mine, and as are the plants and all things that are at one with your nature."

"I feel you still wish to criticise; I feel you are biding your time before you say the word 'but'."

"You read me as though I were your sister rather than your wife. I suppose it is our years together. I suppose I would never be able to surprise you now. Yet you have surprised me this day. I did not imagine that you could create such a masterpiece- so unique- so imaginative- so new."

"But..." he said, reminding her that he was still owed a criticism amongst all this praise.

"But why are there only two people?" Lucy asked, genuinely confused as though his decision was obviously wrong. Only two people and so much space for more. It seemed a waste to her, that the best part of this was minimised by there only being two.

"There will be more!" he laughed, taking Lucy's hand. He was relieved at the observation, expecting a much worse reaction, and to something that it might be too late to change. But it had always been his intention to make more than two people in this, his greatest work of art. It was a good thing that Lucy also desired him to make more.

"I'm sorry," she smiled at him apologetically, reaffirming a trust between them. "You have worked on this solidly for six days, and you have produced so much in that time, I should let you rest."

"I will rest today Lucy," he smiled back, "I always meant that the seventh day would be that on which I rest. But we will see what happens after that. My Adam, and my Eve, they will make more people I'm sure. My world will grow and change, and we will watch it through everything. He will desire to create as I have done. She will desire to make those creations beautiful and judge them as have you. You will see, this will be the making of us, this will make us Gods."

A Moment Gone

Wonderland

The party is so strange. Just a gathering of people in one house, there, told to have a good time. But I can't get out of the bathroom, staring into the mirror. I've never been so beautiful or so soft. I've never seen before. My ears have never heard the music so clearly, I can and want to hear nothing but those songs, over and over.

The first time I was nervous, as every child is nervous of the world as it grows and sees it from a whole new perspective. I didn't want to take anything that would change my perspective on life, but once I'd seen that world I never wanted to go back.

So I stumble down the stairs into the waiting throng that is my friends... 5 people seems like 50. There are people everywhere, but I need them all. Out into the black, colourful night...

"Catch a star with your eyes and watch as it moves slowly towards you and becomes a plane" I always used to do that, lying on the road as if the tarmac were a soft duvet, looking up into a darkness that goes on forever. That could drive you mad, thinking of that, thinking how there is no end, how small we are. If I stopped my mind from wandering it might stumble into fear. I might realise that a car could come, and it might run straight over my body... I give a thought to how that might feel and how fucked up it would be for the others there with me. They always said that lying there was stupid, but they were still giggling about it, noises somewhere distant from my ears. And I would just lie there.

S. Westwood

We saw a UFO once, flashing lights in a big circle flying silently over our heads, just skimming the trees. Maybe that's when they fly, in the small hours when others are oblivious to their own existence, not to mention the existence of others. Maybe we really saw something that night but we will never know. Maybe our consciousness had only just begun. Isn't it a wonder?

A Moment Gone

Man's Fate

"I have not long for this world, so let me tell you of the events that have brought me here, to this bed, my bed of death. For as surely as I lay here I can now claim that I have learnt one of life's secrets- that man does, in fact, have control over his own fate. I am so happy to be dying because this is the conclusion to all my work. I cannot expect you to understand, but you will, and you will understand how this is the result. The fact that you stand there now is how I can believe in my achievement. You are alive as clearly as I die, but why should that be so? Because I have made it such, because I have controlled my destiny, that is how. You are my brother, my twin, but how can you explain that two identical beings have lived such different lives?"

"Because no one is identical David. We look alike, I know, to the point of being duplicates, but our personalities are practically opposite. I love life, yet here you are because you have never been able to love it as I do. I have tried to help you David, and I have failed."

"Don't hurt yourself over this Mathew, this is what I wanted, this is my choice. You are wrong that we were different- I shared all your loves, all your hates, and all your passions."

"David, please calm down and rest, you are ill."

"Yes, I am, and rest is what I should do, and my body barely allows me to do anything else, yet I have to struggle against that which I should do, because I always have, and will do till the end."

"I'm not sure what you are trying to tell me David, perhaps the fever is upsetting your mind?"

"You think I am crazy? Most pioneers and geniuses were thought to be mad at first..."

"I only mean that you should not be troubling yourself. Please rest."

"I will be resting soon enough, but first I have to tell you everything, I have to explain...Write this down Mathew, write my words."

"Say what you need then brother."

"We were born alike, identical, and for all our childhood we played with the same toys and wore the same clothes. We liked the same flavour ice cream and laughed at the same TV shows. But as soon as I had grown a mind to think, this idea came to me, and it took over my entire life. I resigned myself to living this way and living for this one reason only. The idea was my reason to live, but how many men can say that they actually have a reason to live at all? But this was my idea- to prove that I could take control of my destiny- to prove that I did not have to be a mere copy of you, or a copy of any human at all.

"Remember your first love, Emma?"

"Of cause; you hated her."

"I loved her. I loved her more than you ever thought you did. In my mind I could have married her all those years ago. I thought about her every moment of my miserable existence. And before she was with you she had made it clear to me that I could have her- that I was her first choice- yet I cast her into your arms."

"Why?"

"To prove that, no matter what fate hands

you, you can choose your own path. To prove that man can fight destiny.

"I applied for all the jobs that you did, and if they were offered to me, I turned them down. The exams I took, the subjects that we both excelled in commonly, I failed them to break the cycle of our similarities. I had to prove that our paths could be different."

"If this is true David, I am so sorry, none of us knew what you were doing to yourself. If I had known, I would have helped you, and you wouldn't be here."

"Ah, that brings us to here doesn't it? Well it struck me that the best way of proving I could control fate would be to decide for myself when it be my time to die.

"I started with the smoking. For so long I hated the taste and the smell of cigarettes as much as you did, yet I smoked all the same. I would have smoked myself to death if I had been patient enough. But then came the idea of suicide, and my attempts to end my life before my allotted time.

"I cut my wrists, I was saved. I was to jump from my tower block, yet you came to my home and saved me from that. I began to think that I had been given my answer, that man really does not have a choice. But this time I have truly proved it once and for all. My friend found me, but it is too late, I am here, I am dying from the poison of a hundred pills, and not even the doctors can turn my fate back around."

Mathew began to cry pitifully, while his brother smiled triumphantly back at him.

"We knew you needed help, but if only we

had guessed the reasons for this...I am so sorry David."

"But I am not sorry, I die for my purpose, I have my proof."

"But what David? What have you proven? What if misery was your destiny? What if it was your fate that you live like this? Why do you think you lived like this? This was the fate of my brother. David. what if this really was your time to finally go?"

A look of terror took over David's countenance, and the next moment, he died.

A Moment Gone

Little Bird

The little bird had never fit in with the others. They were all so pure of colour- each one of them, perfectly brown and each one the same. How she stood out from them all with her colourful feathers that mimicked the brightest of nature's hues. Blue feathers like that of the Caribbean sea. Green feathers like the brightest summer grass. Yellow like that of the glowing sun. Red like the rose, and her breast, white as the angelic clouds.

The other birds seldom spoke to her, and she was lonely, and alone. She was so far from them, and they never knew her. So when he came, he with his feathers so coloured, she thought that, at last, her life might be changing.

"Come with me over the sea." He had said. "Come to where I live and live a new. There you will find things are different."

She was so taken with him- he that spoke to her as if she were not so strange, that she said she would go. She would make that trip across the sea, and she would go to him. But she was not used to such a journey, and she could not keep up with the pace of his wings. Over the sea she flew, yet now he was gone, and she was flying blindly on, panicking that she would soon tire and crash into the water. But on she went, remembering his words that things would be different, and hoping that what he said was true.

Days and nights she had flown, but now she was flying over land, and now she could stop and rest. Tired and confused from the journey and the things in her mind, she landed her weary body upon one of those dirty grey buildings and looked at her new surroundings.

This was nothing like the place she had come from, that much was true. There were no open fields. There were no sandy beaches. The only nature was caged by fences as though the trees were exhibits in some strange zoo. But she had made it, and he would be there, somewhere, waiting for her.

And so she waited. She sat with the wind rushing through her feathers and she waited. She waited full of hopeless hope. And she watched the other birds as they flew past or landed near by. She watched and she saw that they were all the same, but not the same as her. And even when she decided to fly a while, she saw nothing different. Over towns and over houses, over factories and office buildings, she flew, and she saw. Yet all around her were the grey birds, and he was nowhere to be seen. Nowhere was there one with her colours… Blue as the centre of a flame. Green as the fully clothed tree. Yellow like a buttercup. Red as the setting sun, and her breast, the purest white like waves crashing at the shore.

Occasionally the grey birds would talk to her. Occasionally they would ask her of where she came from. But although they spoke as if they wanted to know her, none of them ever did. She was still lonely, and she was still alone. She had begun to resign herself to it all now. She realised that her life may always be this… that she would always be different… For what could she do to change what was?

A Moment Gone

One day, after she had spent weeks in such a state, she stared down at herself in a puddle on the pavement. Why, she thought... Why was she so different to those other birds? Why was she such garish colours compared to every other bird that flew? Why was she not grey or brown? And as she thought, she heard the distant beating of wings, and she saw the shadow of a hundred birds in the dirty water.

"Hey... come join us."

She heard one of them say, and she looked up at them, shocked to have been spoken to at all.

"Come... we are all traveling home now."

And there she saw a beautiful sight... all those birds... all those beautiful colours.... Blue like the skies in July. Green as an emerald. Yellow like pure sand. Red as a succulent strawberry, and their breasts, white as the newly fallen snow.

She watched them all, she watched as they flew past her, and she watched as each one of them was lost into the distance.

S. Westwood

Wait for the night,
But when it comes it is taken by sleep.
Wait for a 'happy time',
But it makes the plain times feel worse.

Wait for love,
But love ends, and its taste is bitter.
We are waiting for death,
But then there is nothing left to wait for.

A Moment Gone

The Mayor of St Stephens

John Syer was the mayor of St Stephens- a quiet little town where nothing much happened. A town that was always dull and in which the flowers never wanted to grow. It made him so sad to wander out and see the few people of his little community walking about the place with such blank faces, never even bothering to look at their surroundings as they made their way through each day. But then, there was not so very much to see. The houses all looked the same, the gardens were bare, the streets were grey and even the sky was colourless.

The sun never really shone in St Stephens. Although there was a sun, it only ever came out enough to give off some light. No one ever felt the warm touch of its rays or saw the glowing beauty of its glare. Winter and summer were both very much the same, and John welcomed neither.

Being mayor of this austere little town would have been a completely thankless task if it was not for the fact that everyone loved him. No one ever complained and no one ever past him without a courteous greeting. He was respected, and the people of the town would always say that, although the town had its faults, John was certainly not to blame himself.

"It's been a bad year for fruit again hasn't it?" he said to the man whose market stall was practically empty.

"Its not been good," the man replied with a shrug, "but I expect next year will be better, and the fruit I have had has been fresh and tasty."

John smiled, presuming the man was simply trying to spare his feelings, and he went on his way.

He walked to the church, and there he saw the vicar sitting on the stone doorstep.

"Not doing a service today vicar?" John asked him.

"No one comes," the vicar said a little glumly, yet his round face was fixed in a warm smile. "Never mind," he went on, "the people don't need to be here, for God is here is he not? And he is always with the people."

John could only think that if no one went to the church anymore, it must mean that they had all lost their faith. It made him sad, but how could he blame them when they lived in a town that seemed to completely shun the light of the lord?

Feeling all the more sorry for himself, John said farewell to the vicar and went on his way.

Lost in his own solemn thoughts he wandered so far that he reached the outskirts of the town. Up to the top of a yellow-grassed hill he had walked, and there he could see for miles. He could look back and see the dullness that engulfed his town, or he could look forwards and see the rays of sun breaking through the cloud, shinning like beacons down onto the bright little town of St Christophers. How glum it made him to see that difference, and for a moment he thought of walking on and leaving St Stephens forever.

Just as those thoughts came to him a stranger appeared at his side. He knew every face from his own town, and he had never seen this man before. The man was young, yet looked old for his years. His face held a countenance that seemed

A Moment Gone

like pain and his hair was white grey. He was looking at John with a longing gaze that was close to desperation. John presumed that the stranger must be a beggar and it was true enough that his clothes, once perhaps fine, were tattered as rags.

Poor fellow, John thought. The stranger may once have been rich and successful with happiness and youthful beauty, yet something must have befallen him and changed his fate to this. John felt compassion for the man, and decided that he should speak.

"Dear fellow," John said, "is there something I can do for you? I am the mayor of St Stephens."

"I know," the man said, "and I was thinking that perhaps we could help each other."

"Go on..."

"I have something to offer you, a gift, if you will take it," the man said, and he placed one hand deep into the pocket of his coat. "It has been my burden, yet it could be your sweetest saviour."

The man brought his hand back from his pocket and held it out flat in front of John. In his palm there sat a little clear red stone, almost like coloured glass, and shaped like a heart.

"Take it from me," the man said, "but only if you wish it."

"But what is it for?" John asked.

"Have you ever wished that everything in your town was better, was wonderful? Have you never said to yourself, 'I wish the sun would come out for once?'" The man began, his eyes lighting up with his words. "As mayor of St Stephens, have you never wished that your town could know a wonderful summer? A summer where the sun shines each day, where beauty grows and all your people are happy? Have you ever wished that the spirits of your people could be so lifted that they were all filled with joy at the very prospect of being alive? Have you never wanted that?"

"Well of cause," John said wearily, a little confused, "but what are you saying?"

"I am offering you just that," the stranger replied. "This gift, this heart will put the heart into your town. It is my gift to you, it is magic, and it will do just as I said, it will bring a glorious summer upon your town."

John thought on what he had been told, and he realised that he was now to make a decision. For he had no doubts as to the man's integrity.

The man stood there still holding out that heart shaped stone, and John looked at it, thinking of all that it could mean. He thought of the fruit seller with his empty shelves, and he thought of how happy his people would be if, for once, the sun were to come to their town.

"But what happens after the summer?" John said, asking the only question that troubled his mind.

"Everything will be back as it was," the stranger replied, and he held the stone out closer.

"Then yes!" John exclaimed. "I can't lose! Of cause I will accept your gift, thank you."

And with that the stranger tipped his hand and let the stone fall into the hand of the mayor. John clasped it tight and he watched as the stranger silently turned away and began to descend from the hill without a further word.

John felt better already. He felt a flutter of

A Moment Gone

hope in his heart, a hope that the stranger's words would be kept and his town might know some happiness. He did not know if the stone really held some magic, or whether it was just a lucky charm, but he really did believe that it would work and what he had been promised would come to pass.

He smiled to himself that night as he took the stone from his pocket to place it under his pillow. There he lay it gently on the bed and looked at it lovingly. He looked at its perfect shape, which looked like it had been smoothly carved; yet within the clear crimson there was a thin crack that run through the inside.

"Never mind," he said quietly, "do your magic little stone, make my people happy." And he went to bed with the comforting thought that the next day would be a better one- a feeling that he could not remember ever having experienced before.

He was woken, the next morning, by an unusual light shinning right through his curtains and illuminating his entire bedroom. His eyes opened wide, looking around at the bright glow which lit each wall, and then, leaping free of the bed sheets, he pulled back the curtains and beheld what could only be magic!

The sky was clear, crystal blue and the yellow sun was beating gaily down upon his town. Within its warmth his people were walking with skipped steps, literally singing as they went on their way.

Out into the street he ran- to see if it were really true- and there the brilliant reality hit him. It really was as wonderful as he had hoped! And such hope he felt. It seemed like anything was achievable now, that good things could really start to happen.

"Oh John," a woman said in the most light-hearted voice as she made her way past him. "I've never known such a day."

And John had never known such a day either. He had only ever heard that such a thing was possible, but never did he think it would happen in his town!

He felt so happy. In fact, he felt such elation that, for a moment, he thought that he must be dreaming. For everywhere he looked there were people smiling and bathing in the warmth of that sun- a sun that was lighting up everything in the town- bringing colour where once there was grey. Trees were stretching out their branches towards the blue sky and the flowers had opened up to display their beautiful hues. It truly was too wonderful to believe.

He went on his way, walking just to take it all in, and everyone he past greeted him with a huge smile. A man came towards John, walking with his dog. And even the dog seemed to be more content- wagging its tail and practically smiling from its panting mouth.

"I never knew this town could look so wonderful."

John walked all the way through his town and every inch of it had become as beautiful as the next. The houses looked more homely, the gardens were lush with colour and the streets were full of children playing and people simply enjoying their new surroundings. Everyone was carefree and everyone was happy.

John noticed that quite a lot of people were heading towards the church, almost in procession, and so he joined them as they walked.

"Look at this!" the vicar exclaimed. "All these people have come today, to give thanks to the Lord!"

"It is a wonderful magic," John said in awe. And he looked around the church, looking at all the people there, and delighting as they all were, at the way the sun lit up the colours through the stain glassed windows, beaming down and lighting up each pew. It seemed truly believable, in that place, to think that God had blessed them all.

"It was the stone that stranger gave to me," John explained to the vicar. "He gave me a magic stone, shaped like a heart, and it has brought us all such a wonderful hope for the future."

The vicar looked a little concerned, but then he smiled and took John's hand.

"This is your doing?" he asked excitedly.

"Yes," John said, "I was offered the chance to have all this, and because I love my people, just as you do, I happily took that chance."

With that the vicar led John to the front of his church, and together they climbed the few steps to the pulpit.

"Our mayor," the vicar announced, and all the people clapped. "Our mayor has done all this for us- he has performed this magic, and the Lord has provided!"

There was much clapping and talking amongst the congregation, everyone delighting in what they had just heard and giving their thanks. John felt wonderful. He felt loved, happy, and completely filled with joy. He felt things he never thought he would be blessed to feel in his entire life. John felt truly alive.

It seemed that everyone in the town began to live that day. In the weeks that followed the streets were busy with people happily going about their days. The market was overflowing with fresh fruit and vegetables to sell, and heaving with people who wanted to buy it. Even the folk of St Christophers were leaving their town to spend time in St Stephens, and the houses that had been up for sale so long were soon taken up. Life had come to St Stephens- life and light and happiness.

Then it was over.

One day John woke and the light had simply gone from the sky. Out in the street his people were all crowded together with confused and anguished faces, staring up at the grey clouds and looking all about them. They could not believe what they were seeing. And they could not bear the sinking feeling that they all felt in their hearts.

The streets were grey, the houses all looked the same with their gardens bare of colour. No more did the sun shine down with that glowing beauty. No more did the fruit grow ripe on the trees. No more did the flowers choose to grow. And no more did the people smile, or sing, or skip. All the life and all the splendor was lost.

John slowly opened the door of his house and with a growing ache in his heart he went outside.

"What has happened to our town?" a man

said to him.

"This is your fault," a woman accused him.

"Yes, what have you done?" said another. "Your magic has destroyed our town- look at it!"

John looked, and John saw, and he was crushed. Yet despite how awful it seemed, there was something very familiar about the way the town appeared to him.

By then the vicar had made his way into the centre of the crowd, having abandoned his empty church, and his face was now fixed in a grimace like John had never seen on his old friend before. The characteristic smile was no where to be seen.

"I have lost my faith," the vicar said as he bowed his head to the floor. "It is no use pretending. The Lord giveth and the Lord taketh away..."

John felt the heaviness of his heart push a tear from his eye.

The people hate me, he thought. The love has gone from them. And he began to weep as the people wept, and the people stood there, lost and hopeless.

Amongst the throng, John suddenly spotted a face he recognised as that of the stranger. The man that had given him the stone heart was standing amongst his people in fine clothing and with a smile on his youthful face.

"You!" John called out, and the stranger took a pace forwards to address the mayor.

"Yes John Syer?" the man said with a smirk at the side of his pouting mouth.

John reached into his pocket and pulled out the stone. He looked at it for a moment. He looked at the crack that ran through it and saw that it had got worse, it looked broken.

"This," John cried, "this has destroyed our town. This has given my people a fleeting happiness and left them bitter. This has brought us all this pain. You have tricked me."

"I did nothing of the sort," the man said. "I gave you just what I promised. My gift brought your town a glorious summer."

"But I remember asking you," John pleaded, "that after the summer, what then?"

"And I told you the truth," the man replied. "Everything is back as it was."

A Moment Gone

Some Things Hurt You

An angel sat on my shoulder- looking conspicuous. People were beginning to stare. I would like to say that it did not bother me, but it is hard being the butt of people's jokes. I have always been used- taken advantage of- and seen to be unusually sensitive, and somehow different. But my angel was beautiful, and I would not change.

The thugs on the corner saw the angel instantly and one of them crossed the street to where I was walking. I quickened my pace.

"Wait up mate" he wined behind me, but the 'mate' was far off an endearment. How much more could that word have been so turned on its head and spat with such malice? My feet moved faster, but something prevented me running. And he caught me up and stood in front of me.

"Hey I said wait..." he practically shouted into my face and pushed my chest sharply with the palms of his hands. He had taken up the position now, the one that said he was going to hurt me, and that I was his victim.

But on his shoulder, where I expected to see a devil, sat an angel just like mine- yet his angel was dark of eyes and matted of hair. His angel looked tired and dirty. I could tell that he would have given anything to swap with me, but as he could not, he was here, and he was doing this...

Behind me the other two thugs had come to stand, arms crossed, ready to bar my escape. I knew it was useless. I had to prepare myself for what was going to happen. And although I was sick with nerves, and my heart beat fast and heavy, my angel still smiled. And as his fists hit my face- his angel wept.

A Moment Gone

Here It Begins

I awake on the cliffs. The sea roars beneath me and crashes on the rocks. Rocks like giant statues of unearthly beings reaching outstretched arms above the waterline. The sea white and ferocious as it throws its drenched hands against the coast. Well let all that go on, let nature be so full of life, just don't expect it from me. If I had rolled in my sleep I might have fallen, a few hundred feet to an instant violent death. Perhaps I wanted the waters to take me in. Perhaps I wanted to belong to something.

My sleep had brought me no release as I wake to the same mind, this same rejected body. The cans of high strength cider litter around me, a reminder of my inner anguish, if, indeed, I needed one. I am alone and that much is certainly true, the memories coming slowly creeping into my conscious. I would always be alone now. She still deep in my thoughts as much as if she were here with me, yet I know that she would never, truly, be 'with me' again. Every memory, good and bad, every thought of her like needles pushing the nerves of my brain.

I try to stand but my limbs are too stiff. There are more cans and something else behind me but I cannot move my head to see what it is. I think, trying to remember but my memory is hazy. I am paralyzed yet I do not panic. So what if I can't move? Where would I go? Only one thing makes sense and that is the incredibly strong urge to die.

But if I can't get up how am I to throw myself down upon the rocks? Now I am sober how will I get the courage? I hear them calling me, they keep calling me, cries of pain, of my pain, the pain of having nothing.

"It's me, I just can't do this anymore."

"What do you mean it's you? It's me your hurting."

"I didn't mean to hurt you, I, I just can't do this."

My memory cruelly returns. All my senses are alive yet still I cannot move. I hear the sea, I see the sky, and I smell a stench that is both sweet and vile. Those words she spoke will never get old, they will keep on repeating and will never mean so much as they mean right now. She was gone, she doesn't want me anymore. Gone but not forgotten.

Suddenly I am aware of voices, they are near and sound alarmed. They come clearer, the voice of a man, an urgent voice, then the scream of a woman, a voice I recognise.

They get nearer by the second and, again, I try to stir my aching bones. I have no luck. I still cannot move. And I hear that female voice again and I know without doubt that it is her. I thought I would never hear those sweet sounds again, that's why I did what I did. Now that sweet voice is tainted and full of anguish.

"Oh my God what's he done?"

There is movement around me. Black figures fuss around me. Why can't I move? Perhaps I am not awake yet. Perhaps I am trapped in a dream. Perhaps I am doomed to dream forever, seeing and hearing the same things that I see and hear right now. This certainly has the hallmarks of a dream, of a nightmare.

A Moment Gone

"Oh no. It's my fault, because I left him, because of you."

And then I realise. She left me for him, for the man that now holds my wrist to check for a pulse. He puts an ear to my chest and I know what he will hear.

Yes, you did this to me, it *is* your fault. And here I lay, watching this play out before me unable to make a sound or move a limb. I will never move again. I am gone. But a suicide can never escape. Suicides live as I do now, abandoned and forsaken. Forever I will lay incarcerated in a body that responds to nothing, in a mind very much alive with hideous thoughts. They will bury me and I will lie there. They will hold a funeral and from the darkness of my coffin I will hear them speak to me, speaking kind words as though I were still there to hear it. How little they know, and how little I can do about it. I am a suicide. Denied entrance in to heaven, and to hell, doomed to see what I have done and think on it forever more. To go insane trapped in my head.

I remember it all now. Behind me is the mess that ended me, the spoon, the needle I used to dull the pain. Perhaps I knew I had taken too much? But I thought it would give me the courage to jump, instead it poisoned me to death. And that is how it happened, that has been my fate. I am dead, it is over, and here it begins.

When is Now?

Chocolate cake and iced finger buns,
Liquorice wheels and Haribo gums,
A kiss and a hug from the one that I love,
I'm sorry, I'm ill and it's just not enough.

Good films, good music that fill up my soul,
Can't quite fill the void or replace what life stole.
Romance and sex with the one that I love,
I'm sorry, it's selfish, but it's just not enough.

So why am I waiting when I have it all here?
And why is contentment a thing that I fear?
I love her, she's perfect and everything's fine
So why don't I want it, this life that is mine?

If she gave me the word then I would go now,
Holding each other's hands as we fulfill our vow.
To be together forever but not in this life,
And I will be taking an angel as wife.

A Moment Gone

The Brochure

"So I'll leave you for a while and let you make your choice." She said, smiling through her bright red lipstick, no change to her eyes, no cracking of that perfect foundation glaze.

"We can choose anything in the brochure?" He asked her, turning to his wife and then back to the lady in front of him.

The lady held out the thick and glossy brochure, a picture of the Earth from space on the cover.

"Well, whatever you can afford of cause." She said. "How much do you have?"

The man took the brochure and then got distracted by the question. "Err, we don't know." He said and again he looked at his wife who now seemed as puzzled as he was. "How much of what?"

"You haven't even found that out and you are planning to go straight away?" The lady seemed a little put out but the couple had no idea what was going on. "I'll find out for you then," she said, short of patience but hiding it through a professional air. "You just have a look through there, see what you fancy and then we'll find out what your budget is."

"Ok."

And she left them in the white office, all alone. It was silent in there as the couple stared at each other with worried expressions and then stared at the book in the man's hand. They had only been there for a few minutes and already they were experiencing problems. Perhaps once they looked through the brochure they would feel better. Perhaps they could go away together and get back to what they knew and loved.

Their memories were fading, yet they knew that they were important to each other, they knew that they were meant to be as one. But when did they meet? What were their names? He looked at his wife and saw her as he had the first time they ever met. She was beautiful to him, her bobbed brown hair and squared strong face. She was a wonderful person, but just why he knew that he didn't remember. What was a wife? But he knew that she was his.

They sat close and he opened the brochure so that they could both see.

"Mmmm nice looking place isn't it?" He said, looking at the pictures on the first page. He couldn't remember ever being somewhere as perfect as that. It was so green with huge majestic trees and rolling hills.

"I could imagine us there," she said, a familiar voice, comforting and soothing.

He flicked through the first few pages, the wonderful scenery keeping their interest. Then he came to a page where the scenery was even more aesthetically pleasing. White sand stretching out for miles, framed with lush green trees and a turquoise ocean.

"Now that looks lovely," she said, "can we go there?"

"It says it is three thousand credits. What are credits?"

Again the couple shared a puzzled glance.

"It says 'Affluent in Australia. A wonderful

A Moment Gone

experience growing up in a rich family against the back drop of blue oceans and sun twelve months of the year. Rich with wildlife this coastal focused country offers all the comforts of civilisation with the tapestry of the wild.'"

"It sounds expensive," his wife answered.

"Nice though. But how many credits do we have?"

His wife shrugged her shoulders and he turned the pages once more.

At that moment the lady that was serving them came back into the room. She smiled a pearly white grin and cupped her hands.

"You have earnt four hundred credits." She said. "That means that during your life you were not overly mean but you were not completely selfless. You did a few good deeds but generally kept to yourselves. You did not put yourselves out to help people but did not do anyone or anything any harm. Flick to the middle of the book and you will find your choices. Page two hundred onwards."

The man turned over the corners of the book to find the correct page and then he opened it up.

"Horse," he said, reading from the book. "Become a domestic horse used for riding the countryside but generally left alone to graze the pasture land of Cornwall. Three hundred credits."

"Not a bad choice, but there are quite a lot of animals you may be able to afford to be. Take your time, have a look through the brochure and when you have decided what you want to be in your next life give me a shout and we'll sort it out for you. Earth is a good affordable choice but there are plenty of others if you don't find anything you like.

S. Westwood

I'll be out front. Take your time."
Only then did they remember why everything was so familiar yet so unknown. Only then did they realise that they had not survived the crash.

A Moment Gone

Two Souls

All I am is a shell inhabited by blood and bone. My mind is grey mush that somehow sends signals to make my heart beat and my lungs expand when I steal the Earth's clean air. I wonder if you know me, but what is there to know? That I am human, that I have a face and a body...

You have a soul, and it is your soul that I love- your soul that has grown through your life and has not been ruined by the harshness of the world. Your soul is intact.

My life has been a tragedy, a shame, a thing to pity.

Yet your soul glows with innocent light that no tragedy has managed to extinguish, and it always will.

What do you really know of me anyway? You talk as if you know myself better than I. How do you know what I am when I speak so few words to let you into my mind?

You speak to me now don't you?

I have not spoken a word nor opened my mouth all evening.

Yet we speak.

Yes, I suppose we do. I hear your heart as my head rests on your chest, as I cling to you for comfort. And you give me that assurance I so need; I take it from you as sure as I were a vampire. I take the heart I hear and put it with my own.

You have my permission.

And I do not ask twice. I am a limpet here. I will be a fossil with a head lowered to the chest of

S. Westwood

another- four legs and four arms. They will wonder what sort of beast this was, and a brilliant scientist will find the truth someday.

And the beast is love, and together we are one.

A Moment Gone

Stay On These Roads

She past him on her way to the toilets, and he was still there on her way back, slumped on the floor with his knees drawn up to his chest. She had to stop, for he looked so beautiful. He looked like some colourful drawing, as if he were a picture of himself. His hair was jet black and threw itself from its roots in drooping spikes. His face was white and painted dark around the eyes, his cheekbones either distinguishably prominent or also benefiting from well applied make up. His black eyebrows were lowered into a scowl, and his lips were pouted. Yet everything about him had such a prettiness that it did not matter what mood was shown in his countenance.

He made no sign of having seen her, despite the fact that she had stared at him for some time before deciding to speak.

"Hey...Are you ok?"

He did not look up, but spoke into his hands, which rested on his knees.

"It is new years eve, how am I supposed to be happy?"

His voice was moody, and he sounded quite ill at ease, yet she wanted to know more of him.

"What's wrong with new years eve?" She asked.

"Tomorrow is 1990. 1989 will die, and with it goes all the innocence of the eighties. All the androgynous beauty will be old fashioned and reserved for jokes and drag queens. All the cartoon like decadence will be replaced by sleaze. All the unassuming music will drown under a label of what is or is not 'cool'. Sweetness will be lost, or reserved only for children, who can only be children for five years before their adolescence takes over. And all this," he said, throwing a gesturing hand out and waving it about, "all that we now enjoy will be an old man's nostalgia."

She was quite thrown by his emotional outburst, yet quite taken by it all the same.

"How can you possibly say what will happen next year?"

"That's what I like to hear," he mused wistfully, "the innocent, optimistic voice of eighty's youth." He smiled now, allowing his large blue eyes to look up at her so that she saw for certain the chiseled beauty of his made-up features. "Take my word for it," he went on, "if you go on from here you will be dirtied by the whole experience."

There was a pause as she stood there taking in his words and becoming more aware of the music which played on in the hall beyond. Dreamy keyboards were accompanied by the smooth voice of the male singer, unashamed to reach the higher notes usually reserved for the fairer sex.

"Well I hope it doesn't change too much," she started, "but then, things have to move on."

He smiled even wider at her now, with bright white teeth and a cheeky glint in his eyes. "Not always for the better though is it my dear? We should leave it on a high."

She was not sure how to answer anymore, and she felt more than a little saddened at the things he was saying. She stood there and she looked down at her bare arms with her wrists

A Moment Gone

covered in tens of colourful bangles. And she looked at her own white T-shirt with the picture of the group a-ha on the front. She read the words at the bottom which suddenly meant so much more than they ever had before- 'stay on these roads'... And then, in a sudden wave of misery, she slumped down next to the strange boy.

He looked at her with his unwavering smile and put an arm around her back, his long black coat engulfing her and keeping her safe.

"We'll stay here then?" She said.

"Here is best" he nodded.

The hours melted away, and they sat there. For song after song. Dance after dance. Drink after drink. For the entire night they sat there together. And as time past they were joined by one, then another, and another until the entire corridor was full of beautiful, miserable people. They all sat there, and they waited, and when the clock struck twelve, there was not a single cheer.

The Way Past

So this was what I had decided- this was my life. I would dedicate my very existence to the security of this bridge. I would let no one over it- I would protect it and all that was on the other side. I had a purpose, as every demon must have. I was the protector of the bridge. I was the keeper of the borders. If anyone should try to cross this way I would show my sharp, oversized teeth and growl my evil warnings.

"No one shall pass this way unless their reason is fit by me..."

"My reason is to obtain food for my family," the man said, standing, shaking with nerves at the foot of my bridge.

"Why must you go this way?" I asked in an intimidating hiss, "is there no food for you anywhere else?"

"There is food sir," the man stuttered in obvious anxiety, "but not much, and nothing befitting my loved ones."

Fool. To think that I would find this reason worthy. Let them eat what scraps there were. Whether the taste be good or the sustenance fulfilling. I was not going to grant his way past.

"You may not pass this way," I said, and the man obeyed.

I kept my ground, pacing the wooden boards of the bridge and watching the treacherous waters pass underneath. Then, in time, a day came that had me stand firm and say my words:

"No one will pass this way unless their reason is fit by me." I boomed in my best

A Moment Gone

demonesque voice.

"But the one I love is on the other side of this bridge." The man said painfully. I had no desire to grant his wish.

Then, on the other side of me, and for the first time, someone attempted to cross back from the North side.

"Stop!" I called loudly to the pretty girl that walked slowly over the boards of my bridge. "Where do you think you are going?"

"The one I love is there on the other side," she said woefully, "He is right there." And I saw how her eyes fixed on those of the man that stood on the South side, the man that had requested travel over my bridge only moments ago.

"He is your lover?" I asked to make sure.

"Yes," she answered, though she looked only at him.

My glare went from that misty eyed woman and back to the man that took that love so freely. I was struggling with my mind to make a decision as to whether they should be permitted to be reunited with one another or not. But surely my evil should keep them from their wish.

"We are to be married." The man said, his shinning dark eyes melting into those of the girl.

And then I realised... I was a demon was I not? I was an evil creature put on this Earth merely to bring misery upon the human race. Was it not in my very nature to upset the course of love if love was their joy? No. The answer came to me. I made a demon's decision. I would let them come together and over the years I would watch them tear each other apart. Let them live their happy ever after and see that it is flawed. See how long it takes before their love becomes bitter hate. What else could I do that would give me such evil satisfaction?

"Of course you may cross," I said.

A Moment Gone

Your Time Will Come

The apple had no intention of falling from the tree too soon; he liked it just where he was. From a branch that high you could see so much, yet never be seen. From up there you had not got to deal with the chaos of the world below, yet the real world, the beauty of nature, was always at hand. He was part of all that, grown there over the passing months, through the sun and through the rain. He was not ready to go, because he was not ready. An apple has its life cycle just as everything does, and he had not yet seen his moment of glory.

He thought, once, that he had been as great as he could ever be. Once he had been a pretty, delicate blossom, and he could hear how the people spoke of him, and of what pleasure he brought. But one day, he knew that he would be ripe and have that moment of splendor that would make all the hardships fade away into history. All of those hard times, suffering the elements, were making him grow large and perfectly round, green and red, sweet without bitterness. And so when the winds blew, he held on with all his might. When the sun shone, he basked in its light. And he always made sure to drink in the rains.

Children would play below him and he swung proud on his branch, listening to their gentle voices. Yes, he had been like they once; he had been the bud that grew and made the tree so happy to go on each year. They may not notice him now, but one day they will love him, one day he will be known and bring such happiness…

But he was content, that was sure enough.

He was content in his knowledge, the knowledge of good things to come. He was happy to observe all that past him, and all the little pleasures that each day showed him. He loved to listen to those children laughing.

"Mmm, I'd like an apple actually."

He caught a little of their conversation, and before he could understand it, he was caught in the grasp of the little boy's hand. He was plucked, taken from all that he knew, taken from the security of his tree. But maybe this was it…Maybe this was his moment.

A little cherub mouth closed around his skin and took of his being…

"Errr!"

An instant of voiced disgust, and without a pause the apple found himself thrown to the ground, wasted, wounded and finished.

This was not how it should be; this was not his dream. But as the time drifted by his discarded body, as those hardships came once more, the sun tightening his skin and the rain battering him into the ground-he grew from his pain the beginnings of a new hope. He grew and he became a tree.

A Moment Gone

The Gift

He had spent his whole life clutching onto that gift, wrapped in brightly coloured paper, a wonderfully patterned parcel. He knew what it held, he had wrapped it years ago, and he had put his whole self into it, keeping it safe for all those years.

Everyone knew he had it, they saw it and they knew what might be inside. He would even let them hold it sometimes, but after a while he would grow anxious and make them give it back. It was like his baby. Yes you can pick it up, you can look on it, but it is mine. He could never risk any harm coming to it. No one was permitted to open it. It had to remain wrapped.

Until her.

She had never actually asked for the gift, but so taken was he, by her, that he felt compelled, for the first time in his life, to give it away. He truly believed that the gift had always been meant for her.

She smiled at its beautiful paper, she delighted in unwrapping it, and once she had it she held it close against her as though she would never let it go. He had made the right choice and she really seemed to love his gift. So long it had been in his care, but now it was put in her trust alone, and he was pleased. Nothing could have made him any more happy.

Weeks past until, one day, she came to him and she gave it back.

He did not understand and he tried to make her take it. 'It is for you,' he said to her 'I don't want it back, it is for you.' But she just did not want it anymore. And now he held it, opened, discarded, and meant for no one.

As she walked away, as he looked at her fading away from him, he saw something for the first time. She too had a gift, just as his. She clutched it tight, that gift, still wrapped in brightly coloured paper... a wonderfully patterned parcel.

A Moment Gone

You Are Inside

See your face in the mirror
Touch your face with no feeling
The glass lies because that is not you.

Painted face on a canvass
Strokes of brush and colour
Melt in the heat into nothing.

For you are inside
Your clothes are just cloth
Your friends are characters in some obscure film
In which you make a cameo, for a while.

You are inside
So deep inside that you may never find yourself.
Perhaps you should not try.

S. Westwood

A Lemming Thing To Do

For my wife Ashley x

The little lemming walked slowly towards the edge of oblivion... He followed the others... Others he had seen, and others he had known. He followed his friends and his family. He followed and he asked no questions. He was a lemming, this was a lemming thing to do, there were no questions to ask.

He walked on in a straight line, in procession, with those in front leading the way. He walked towards the sound of the sea... to the horizon ahead... towards the clouds.

After he had walked for about ten minutes he began to grow weary and he stopped to rest on a big grey rock, resting his tired lemming feet. While sitting there a black bird landed on the rock beside him and spoke...

"Where are you all going?" He asked.

Well the lemming hadn't given it much thought until now, but he had to answer the bird truthfully, as lemmings never told lies.

"I'm not entirely sure," he said, "I'm just following the others."

"Well I wouldn't go that way if I were you," the black bird said. "I have flown that way and there is nothing to see there but the edge of the cliffs."

"Well aren't the cliffs quite beautiful?" The lemming asked.

"Beautiful? I suppose they are," the bird said thoughtfully. "Well good luck little lemming, I'll bid you farewell," the bird said with a bow, and off he flew.

The lemming got up and went on his way hurrying a little as the procession was heading off without him. He walked on and on, following the others and getting quite tired and extremely thirsty... so when he saw a little stream he decided to stop and have a drink. He lowered his little lemming mouth and he took a drink from the clear water. As he did so a small yellow fish popped out its head and she spoke.

"Where are you all going?" the fish asked.

"Don't really know," the lemming answered, "I'm just following the others."

"Well I wouldn't go that way if I were you," the fish said. "I have swam that way and the waters are deep and rough against the rocks."

"But isn't the sea blue and quite beautiful?" The lemming asked.

"Blue? Yes. And beautiful? I suppose it is," the fish said as she thought on it. "Well good luck little lemming, I'll say good bye." And with that the little fish dived back down into the stream and off she swam.

The lemming left the stream and started back on his way, now hardly able to see those that he followed as they were so far ahead of him. But on he went following the procession until he past an apple tree and there he stopped, realising how very hungry he had become.

As he reached up to try and pluck an apple from an over hanging branch a monkey spotted him and spoke.

"Where are you all going little lemming?"

The monkey asked with a cheeky grin.

"Just following the others," the lemming admitted... "I don't know where we are going."

"Well I wouldn't go that way if I were you," the monkey said. "I have been to the very top of this tree and I can see everything... there are no more trees, just open spaces, nothing that way that is worth all this walking."

"But my friends are all going that way... my family are all going that way... so I have to follow."

"Well if you think so little lemming, I'll say cheeryo for now." And with that the monkey threw down an apple, smiled a huge smile and jumped up to the top of the tree.

"Thank you." The lemming called out, and he sat and he ate the nice juicy apple.

Once he had finished he set to walking again and to his chagrin he realised that he could no longer see the procession at all.

"Oh my," he said to himself and he looked around, jumping up and down in the hope of seeing further. "Oh dear." He said. "Now I won't be able to see those beautiful cliffs or that beautiful sea... now I wont be with all those that I have always known... now I..." And he began to cry. Then he saw the black bird flying overhead and it waved to him with a friendly wing. And the monkey had come down from the tree to see what was wrong. Behind him he heard a splash, he looked around and there, again, was the pretty yellow fish.

"Why are you crying little lemming?" The fish asked.

"Yes, why do you cry?" The monkey said.

And it was only then that the lemming

A Moment Gone

realised that he had made three new friends and seen three new and wonderful places...

"I don't know." The lemming said truthfully, as lemmings always tell the truth. "I was just following the others. I guess I'll just have to follow them some other day."

And with that, the lemming dried his eyes.

A Push Too Far

It all started with throwing sticks from the bridge and watching them fall with a splash into the stream below. He had stolen the idea from an episode of '*Winnie The Pooh*' where all the animals threw 'pooh sticks', watching them catch the current of the water and float away like ships in a breeze. But Sam was not playing with a load of stuffed toy animals; he was not playing with any friends at all, for he did not really have any. He was on his own and, despite the initial fascination, the game soon became boring. Anyway, he did not really get any enjoyment out of watching the sticks drift away in the water, it was just the way they fell that captivated him, and it was always too short a moment.

But when you enjoy something that much, it can often become a habit, and then, after a little longer, it may become an addiction. Sam skipped the habit and went head long into a total obsession. Sam would lie awake in bed, thinking of things he could throw and places to drop them from. Sam would spend his weekends walking around in search of tall buildings that he could access and use for his hobby, (if indeed that is what it was). And he soon bored of throwing sticks and screwed up paper- the things he chose to watch, as they descended out of his hand and down to the ground, had to become bigger and become more unusual.

Sam had a sister, and his sister had a doll. That doll smashing on the tarmac after a slow tumble over the wall of the multi-storey car park was on Sam's mind for weeks before he managed

A Moment Gone

to smuggle it out of the house and fulfil his fantasy. The moment lasted for only seconds, but his sister cried for weeks.

He knew that he had to find an answer to all this- something to quench the thirst- to feed the hunger. He knew he was mad, he knew it was not normal, but if he could just find something that satisfied him, then he could live with this compulsion.

As it turned out, his family moved, of cause, taking Sam with them, and that was when he set eyes on the quarry. Sam had never even dreamt of a place like this- a place where he could spend hours playing his favourite game in solitude and undisturbed. There was all the height he needed and all the rocks he could ever want for the purpose of throwing them down the pit and watching them drop. This would be his playground, and he could not remember ever being so excited before.

Sam's family had turned a blind eye to his strange behaviour up till now. The fact that he knew he was strange seemed to make it a little more acceptable. Yet they began to worry when he spent entire days at the quarry for no other reason but to throw rocks over the side. It was just not a normal thing for a child of ten to be doing, or for anyone to do as it happened. It was plain weird.

"When are you going to get over this Sam?" His father asked him one day.

"I don't know, I mean, I enjoy it."

"But you could be doing so many other things Sammy."

"I just like pushing the rocks, I like seeing

them break, you know, and thinking about things. I like watching them fall, and it helps me to think about things all the more."

"You're only ten Sam, you shouldn't think so much."

But no conversation stopped Sam from what he was doing, because each rock he pushed gave him pleasure.

The first time he had thrown a rock over into that quarry he had almost burst with the excitement of it. Yes, he had thrown things before, but this was special, even better than the doll. This went far, this was beautiful. It crashed at the bottom and shattered into pieces. And for the times that followed, he got a repeat of that joy and he remembered the joy of the first, and he was so happy. But time changes things. It was almost as if the quarry bored of him, and it stopped supplying him with the joy it had once given so freely. Every rock seemed to fall faster, and without that smash which climactically signalled its end. But no where else was interesting anymore. He threw everything he could find down into that quarry. Toys. Jigsaw pieces, mirrors... oh yes he loved how they smashed, but the rocks were such a perfect object for his affections. And now affection was becoming affliction.

But Sam never gave up in his pursuit for that joy he had once tasted. Sam went on, every day, going to that quarry, pushing those rocks, trying new ways to let them go. But he remained unfulfilled, he continued to be disappointed, and every rock seemed to fall less dramatically. He started to wonder if it would have been better if he

A Moment Gone

had never experienced that long lost elation, for then he would not be missing it so. He began to think bad thoughts. He began to imagine throwing himself off into the pit. If only he could sit and watch himself go. He would have loved to watch someone else do it, yet he had no romantic notions about suicide, only the beauty of that descent- like some great bird swooping for its prey. He knew that there might be a time that the rocks were not enough for him.

He tried, and he tried to get it all back. That elated feeling. He tried so hard that he did not even realise what was happening, and what was happening to him. Yes, it was obsession, yes, it was unhealthy, but it seemed so right... And then, one day, he pushed just one more rock and he saw what he had done...

The quarry was full, the rocks were stacked so high that they were spilling over the edge and back towards where he sat. He had done all he could do and he had failed to find that old happiness. There was no going back; he had pushed too far.

S. Westwood

Lay back in the sea. Float on the ripples as they
tease you and move you.
Close your eyes and let the waves lift you up and
carry you away.
Feel the rays of the sun as they reflect on the water
and soak into your skin.
Hear the gentle rush of the tides.
The beauty is happening around you, and you
know it is there...
One day you will reach the island, you will open
your eyes, and you will see where you have been
taken.

A Moment Gone

The Lion Tamer

Ferocious, the master of all beasts and king of the jungle. He scared every animal with his roar, so loud that the very trees shook in terror. He frightened all with his huge fangs ripping through the flesh of a zebra, freshly killed.

"I've never actually seen him kill," Hugo the hyena told his fellow hyenas around the fire one quiet night, "but all the more to fear. His stealth is our enemy."

Hugo was new to the group. He had travelled far from his old pack and no one knew anything about him. Yet he did seem to know a lot about the lion.

"Something should be done about him," one of the youngsters said quickly, as if the speed of its delivery would nullify the words feared to be out of line.

"My point exactly," Hugo went on, "and I'm the hyena to do it!"

"You're going to stand up to him?" asked the eldest.

"In time, in time," Hugo said. "First we must join together."

"Join together?" the elder scoffed.

"Form an alliance!" Hugo exclaimed. "And we need a name. All of us must go away and think of a name."

"Ok," the youngster said enthusiastically.

"A name," the elder said looking around at his fellows, "is that all?"

"It is" Hugo said. "Together we will face this menace."

The next night the hyenas grouped around the fire as usual, but they were all more excited than usual and noisily discussing the day.

"Did you see him today?" Hugo asked rhetorically. "I saw him, the almighty lion, prowling close to our homes. We must be on guard. I will appoint everyone a duty. But first- the name!"

The elder looked at the others and a worried expression took over from his all knowing countenance.

"Yes, ok," he coughed. "I think I know what we should be called, but does anyone else have a name for our, our..."

"Alliance!" Hugo finished.

"How about, The Fangs" one of the hyenas spoke up.

"The Secret Claw," a young one announced.

"The Lion Tamers" the elder said quite sure of himself.

"That's it," Hugo said. "And you will be Chief of Police against the lion threat."

The elder lifted his nose a little as if so doing was the beginning of his duty.

"You there" Hugo pointed. "You will be look out for the night, a very important job. And you," he pointed to another, "you will be look-out tomorrow."

He then went on to appoint a Chief Investigator, a Captain, a scribe to keep log and each hyena was to be called a Private in the army of the 'Lion Tamers'. Each had their very own duty and all felt very important and couldn't believe how long they had allowed the lion to rule the kingdom unchallenged.

A Moment Gone

The next night every hyena in the 'lion tamers' joined together to talk again about the rebellion and catch up on news about the almighty lion.

"He was swaggering in our patch," the look-out said, "as if he hadn't a care in the world."

"The nerve of it," said captain one.

"Something must be done," the elder said.

"In time, in time," Hugo said. "First we need a uniform."

"Yes we should have one," a few said in unison. All seemed quite fired up at the prospect.

"War paint," the elder said.

"Indeed," Hugo answered. "Tomorrow we will group by the water hole and draw on each other with the red mud. We will look truly menacing."

And so they did just that. Each hyena was sure that the war paint made them look ready for a fight. They were fired up. But Hugo did not order them to attack. "All things in good time," he said, "we need a song."

"Of course," one of the females said. "Hugo is right. All armies chant. We need a chant to take us in to battle!"

All looked to Hugo for orders. He had soon become the most important of all their group and the leader of the 'Lion Tamers'. Everyone commented that they did not know how they had coped without him. Even the eldest admitted to being glad Hugo had come to them.

"You are a brave and noble beast," the elder said, "we trust you to provide us with a song."

Hugo said he would need a day to write it and ordered that they group together the next evening to learn it. As the sun turned red on the horizon all the hyenas came together and started the fire as they did every night. The temperature dropped as the sun ceased its glow and last to arrive was Hugo.

"I have it," he said, and the others cheered. And Hugo took up an animated stance, his whole face lighting up with his genius.

"Fearsome beast with large teeth, we are not afraid, we are not afraid.
Lion strong, lion fierce, we are not afraid, we are not afraid. And I have come to lead you on, we are not afraid, we are not afraid.
Now nothing will be the same for we will lion tame, lion tame."

Hugo finished with hands to the darkening sky and everyone clapped and wailed.

"It is perfect!" One of them said and all agreed.

"From this day we will train and learn the song." Hugo said. "We will be as one!"

And a cheer went up in to the night. Weeks went by. They watched out for the lion. If he made an appearance they were all sure he was up to no good. If they did not see him at all they were sure he was planning something. Hugo taught them all to march, to chant their song and taught them all he knew about lions. So many things were new to them. For instance, they had no idea that lions could jump from the top of trees on to their prey. It was for this reason that some of the hyenas were posted at the top of trees to look out.

A Moment Gone

"Thank God you came to us," they said, "it is a weight lifted." But it wasn't. If they could really see what was happening they were now more paranoid about the lion than they had ever been before. Some of them were getting itchy for a fight.

"We can't let that lion go on like this," the elder said, "it's time we made our move."

"In time," Hugo said, two words he had used over and over. "He is a ferocious beast, and we are weak."

"Are we not strong now?" one challenged.

"Yes. We are an army now, let us fight!" Another said.

"In time," Hugo insisted.

They trusted Hugo completely and the lion was incredibly scary so perhaps it was right that they go on with their training. Learning the song, practicing the war paint... Hugo was a God send to the pack. Before he came they had been unorganised and just let that lion do what ever it pleased. No more would they take it.

"You said he killed ten zebras and didn't even eat them."

"You said he was training his pack to fight us. Shouldn't we do it now, before he gets them organised?"

"Let's do it, tomorrow!"

Hugo tried again to calm them down but they had ceased listening.

"We are ready. Don't you feel ready?"

"We are ready," the elder said. "Tomorrow it is. At sun up we will group up and we will fight!"

It had come about sooner than he wished but

they were going to do it, with or without him. That night he said that he would be the watch man. The hyenas slept and Hugo had only the hours of darkness to get away. He wasn't crazy. There was no way he was going to stand up to a lion. Even with them all together some would be bound to die and Hugo was certain he would not be one of them. So, once he was sure that all eyes were from him he tiptoed out of the den with his few possessions in a sack. The fire had almost gone out, a few red embers lighting the path that was his exit. Hugo would miss them but he would have to find another pack to join. He would have to start it all over again.

He had not travelled far before he saw the lion on the path ahead. He froze in terror. The lion was eating a zebra, grinding bones with his teeth and ripping at the flesh with his fangs. Hugo watched, impotent with fear, and the lion looked up meeting his eyes. Hugo's legs became useless and the lion need only pounce and he would be gone. The lion growled, snorted, and then spoke.

"I'm finished here," the great beast said, "would you like to finish it off?"

Hugo laughed. It was in relief and in utter dismay.

"What?" was the only word he could muster.

"The zebra," the lion said, "would you like the rest?"

"Why yes." Hugo said and went tentatively closer. The lion smiled and despite his vicious teeth looked perfectly benign. Hugo ate and the lion went down to the water to drink. Hugo could not relax, one eye on the lion, one on his supper.

A Moment Gone

The meat was good. But the lion did not go away and Hugo wondered if it was just biding its time before killing him. Yet as he joined the lion at the water hole the lion smiled again in what could only be described as genuine kindness.

At the water's edge a terrible splashing heralded the attack from a hungry alligator. Its great jaws took hold of Hugo and the creature began to drag him down into the water. Behind him he heard an almighty roar and before long he was free from the 'gator's grip and struggling for breath in the water's shallow edge. He was in great pain and losing a lot of blood. He lay in the mud and his eyes refocused. The lion was fighting the alligator. It was saving him, fighting for him and without much effort the lion had seen off the threat.

"Are you badly hurt?" The lion asked gently.
Hugo tried to form words but he was finished, the alligators teeth had pierced through his flesh. Blood was pouring out from him and turning the dark water red around him. The lion pushed Hugo's dying body out of the water and further on to the bank.

"Hyena... are you ok?" The lion asked urgently.

If Hugo could speak there would be a thousand things to say. If he was to live this lion would have saved his life. The lion he had persecuted for his own selfish purpose. This creature he had used to the death to enhance his own pointless status. It was his doing that at morning light the other's he had made his friends would execute his saviour. If only he could talk, if he could warn the beast, say a thousand times sorry. But as the words stuck in his throat the last breath came and Hugo, leader of the 'Lion Tamers', leader of a bogus unjust fight, died.

A Moment Gone

Timetable

He slowly lowered himself down the embankment, holding onto clumps of grass, his boot digging into wet dirt. But so what if he fell? So what, so what?

It was dusk, so not yet too dark to see. There was a gentle, silent sheet of dark grey cloud thrown over the sky. Everything seemed that little more beautiful in that half-light. Everything was hidden from harshness, and everything seemed benign. The green grass was glowing blue, and the train tracks below were a soft, shinning purple. Who would have guessed? Who? Who would have guessed?

He was down there now, standing just behind one of those metal tracks.

He looked to the right, where the tracks went on and then curved out of sight. That was where the train would come from. He had planned this. There would be no chance of failure, not this time. No, not this time...

He had used pills before, but he was found, and he was taken to hospital. He was lucky, they said, for he had not taken enough to be fatal. And before that it had been his wrists. He had cut into his arms with a blade, but although the cuts were deep, they only bled in drips, and it would have taken weeks. This time he would not end up in hospital. This time it would take less than a second. This time he would do it right...

He wondered, as he stepped out onto the track and into the middle. He wondered if, even for an instant, he would feel the pain. It was bound to be quick, exploding into fragments at over one hundred miles an hour, but would he feel it? What would he feel?

A distant clattering sound hailed the coming of the end. A white light moved slowly around the curve and was now coming down the tracks. It was coming. The 6.15 to London. The train, and the end was on its way. His watch said 6.18, perhaps the train had been late? Perhaps it was not too late?

There was time to change his mind, but he wished that there was not time. He wished that it was more inevitable. Yet he was not moving was he? He did not panic enough to move. The panic was controlled, and as the train grew closer he only felt more comfortable.

Yes, this is it... This is your time... Grit your teeth, close your eyes, bury your face in the palms of your hands, think of nothing, hear your heartbeat for the very last time...

That noise, that deafly noise...

That sound, that deathly sound...

And it had gone.

He stood there, raising his head now, opening his squinting eyes, and allowing himself to look behind at the tracks on which he stood. And there, there in the distance, the train was moving away.

No, not his time, not this time. Better check the timetable.

www.ingramcontent.com/pod-product-compliance
Lightning Source LLC
Chambersburg PA
CBHW031207270326
41931CB00006B/450